Sexual Ecstasy & the Divine

Sexual Ecstasy & the Divine
The Passion & Pain of Our Bodies

Yasmine Galenorn

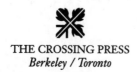

THE CROSSING PRESS
Berkeley / Toronto

The Crossing Press
www.crossingpress.com

A division of Ten Speed Press
P.O. Box 7123
Berkeley, California 94707
www.tenspeed.com

Library of Congress Cataloging-in-Publication Data on file with the publisher.

ISBN 1-58091-113-7

Cover design by Nina Miller
Text design by Jeff Brandenburg/Image-Comp.com
Front cover photo by Suza Scalora/Getty Images

First printing, 2003
Printed in the United States

1 2 3 4 5 6 7 8 9 10—08 07 06 05 04 03

High sex takes the experience of orgasm to a new dimension—a dimension in which genital orgasm is only the beginning. It inspires you to explore the full capacity of orgasm, culminating in ecstatic body-to-body and soul-to-soul experiences in which physical pleasure becomes a delight of the heart and an ecstasy of the spirit.

—Margo Anand, *The Art of Sexual Ecstasy*

Dedicated to

Shiva and Shakti
and
to all women and men who manifest the face of
the Goddess and the God in their unions with
one another and their joy in their own bodies.
This means you.

Acknowledgments

Like its sister book, *Crafting the Body Divine*, this book has not been an easy one to write. Emotionally draining, exhilarating, terrifying at times, it has been quite an experience. I give my deepest thanks to:

My husband, Samwise Galenorn, who has served as a most talented research assistant, and whom I love dearly.

Those who have volunteered to be my research assistants. Some of you may have been quite fun; others—well, it made life interesting to receive your offers.

I also wish to thank:

Joseph, with whom I've had many fascinating discussions on the mentality and mechanics of BDSM and passion.

Offline and online friends who offered emotional support during the writing of this book: Alexandra, Siduri, Lisa, Johnny, Daniela, Sue, Saga, Geoff, and many more.

All my readers who kept asking me when this book was coming out, once they'd heard I was planning on writing it, and who patiently waited through all the delays and snafus that caused this book to be late in reaching the shelves.

Much thanks to Astrid Sandell, for encouraging me to write this book.

As always, I give my deepest love to my Lord and Lady, Mielikki and Tapio, who have lived in my heart over twenty-two years since I've been in the Craft.

The Painted Panther
—Yasmine Galenorn

Contents

Contents

Introduction

Sexual Ecstasy & the Divine and *Crafting the Body Divine* began their existence as a single book. When I changed publishers, instead of trying to edit down the large and rather daunting manuscript, my new publisher offered me another option: why not divide it into two separate books?

While the parts that became *Crafting the Body Divine* felt complete, I hadn't been able to expand on the sexuality sections as much as I had hoped to, primarily because I was running well over a hundred thousand words, which is hard to get published in this genre.

When offered the opportunity to expand my manuscript into two volumes, I immediately jumped at it. Now I could take a subject I love writing about and really explore it as I had originally planned. Hence, we have both *Crafting the Body Divine* and *Sexual Ecstasy & the Divine*—linked and yet separate, much like fraternal twins.

Within the pages of this book, I intend to guide you on a safari of sorts, with the goal of forging a cosmic connection with the gods through the use of your sexuality. I want to help you learn how to enjoy your body and your passion, to help you overcome any lingering embarrassment while striving for divine communion.

To this end, I have provided exercises, frank discussions, and meditations to help you become comfortable with all aspects of your sexuality—from masturbation to intercourse to ritual sex. Sexual-spiritual work requires us to release old habits and let go of any shame embedded within our hearts and minds. We must set aside preconceived notions and biased judgments in order to examine what lies beneath some of our most intimately held beliefs. We must be willing to take a few risks, some of which will remain within the confines of our thoughts. It's not easy, I won't say it is, but if you are willing to take the journey, I will lead you through the maze as best as I can.

Sexual Ecstasy & the Divine explores the connection between sex and spirit, an intersection that is one of the most beautiful and powerful places in the universe.

I include excerpts from my own life. I offer them up to public scrutiny only to help you gauge what you might want to try (or not try) in your own lives. One of the nicest comments I hear from readers is: "It sounds like you're talking to me over a cup of tea." While this is a wonderful compliment, a book like this one explores very personal details in my life. Please respect this fact when, and if, you write to me. I love the feedback I receive from my readers, but among the vast majority of wonderful letters, I've also received a few that were not so wonderful.

So before you contact me, please note the following:

> ❧ **I do not offer personal advice: no exceptions.** I'm not a professional counselor, and I don't have the time, with my writing and my personal life, to help others beyond the confines of this book and the information on my domain (see Galenorn En/Visions at www.galenorn.com for my various websites and contact information).

> ❧ To the very few who have written to me in this vein: I neither need to hear nor want to know your sexual fantasies. Nor do I want to be offered invitations to participate in them in any way. NO. Period. Don't even bother.

Sex is a loaded gun. We use it to sell products, to win friends and influence people. We wallow in it, yet call it sinful. We crave it, yet we fear it. Perhaps, with effort, we can allow sex to be what it truly is: a joyful function of our bodies, a union between people who seek to explore the spiritual through the carnal, a fun romp in the meadow when we're feeling as squirmy as a bunch of frolicking puppies, the cementing of a friendship into a deeper commitment, a bond of love expressed through the body, and, at the core, the divine and holy dance of the God and Goddess as they create life through the universe by way of their union.

Bright blessings, my friends, and may your life be filled with passion.

The Painted Panther
—YASMINE GALENORN

CHAPTER ONE

A Brief History of Civilized Sex

There are those who say my purpose is to demystify the
female body, but that is an impossibility. The female body
will always be a very great mystery, no matter how many
you see or how much knowledge you achieve. You can
never demystify a cervix. It's a magnificent miracle—the
doorway to life itself.

ANNIE SPRINKLE, *Public Cervix Announcement*

Love and sexuality today is not what it was two thousand years ago. When
we examine the beginnings of love and lust, we find that while there were
numerous deities connected with these emotions, interpersonal relationships were pretty bleak in many of the ancient cultures.

Sexual Ecstasy & the Divine is designed to help you free yourself from
guilt and shame about your sexuality. My ultimate goal is to help you discover the spiritual side of passion and sex. We will first take a brief look at
sexuality through the ages, especially the demonization and erosion of
women's sexuality. By denigrating the female sexual nature, many religions
and cultures managed to cast the sexuality of *both* men and women into the
gutter.

Even a quick exploration into the past gives us a solid foundation from which to view the present state of affairs and explains why so many of us were brought up to be ashamed of our genitals and our sexual nature.

Sumer to Judea: The Code of Hammurabi

In ancient Sumer, approximately 2500–1800 B.C.E., conditions for women were a little better than they became later. Though women were considered to be their father's property, life wasn't too bad. Some fathers donated dowries to the temple—which now owned the women—and the women answered to the priests and the gods. Temple women were respected for their work, whether it be as a sacred harlot or priestess. Sumer is the motherland of astronomy and mathematics as we know them today, and most of the discoveries were made among the priests and priestesses, so education did exist for women.

Marriage, well, as with most other cultures throughout time, the woman became her husband's property. However, during this time period, her dowry was bestowed upon both her husband and herself, and was primarily hers to control. The women also retained an equal say over their children, though the children became their father's property.

Punishment for adultery for women was death. A woman who found her husband involved with another woman was entitled to divorce him, and she was eligible to receive child support and custody of the children. No divorce for any reason other than adultery or neglect existed for her. However, a man could divorce his wife whenever he chose.

When Hammurabi, king of Babylon, rose to power and displaced Sumerian rule (1792–1750 B.C.E.), he created one of the first written codes of justice that systematically divided the law into differing subjects. Women's rights began to erode with this new code. Alimony and child support were still awarded to women whose husbands divorced them, but, as in many cultures, women often received punishments far harsher than those given to men.

Women who committed adultery were executed by drowning. Men were punished economically. Women could only obtain a divorce as a result of their husband's infidelity. Laws and punishments regarding various aspects of sexuality began to appear, including a death sentence for incest or homosexuality. Laws also adjudicated where temple priestesses were to live and how they were to behave.[1]

However, life for women was still tolerable and, in many cases, quite pleasant. Women still had the right to become judges, elders, and scribes. They were prominent in the arts and crafts communities, and—when behaving according to society's moral code—were accorded a great deal of respect. Even concubines who conceived were entitled to restitution from the fathers-to-be.

The next period in this area of the world saw a drastic weakening of women's rights to their bodies and their lives. In Mesopotamia, from 900–600 B.C.E., we encounter MAL 40 (Middle Assyrian Law 40): the law regarding the veiling of women. All respectable women were to veil themselves when appearing in the streets (an obvious predecessor to the chador or *burqua* worn by Islamic women). Harlots, temple concubines, slaves, women cast off by men, and freeborn concubines remained uncloaked in an effort to distinguish them from the respectable women: wives, daughters, widows, and concubines of Assyrian businessmen.

This law newly defined women's roles and defined a woman as the sexual and physical possession of a man. When she slept with whomever she chose or committed herself to temple activities, she was considered disreputable. Priestesses fell into the same category as the common whore, an important division that defined how Middle Eastern cultures looked upon women who served the gods.

When we arrive at early Judean culture, we find this subjugation complete. Women were expected to call their husbands *Ba'al* (meaning master),

---

1 See chapter 5: Sheelah Na Gigs and Sacred Harlots, for more information.

or *Adon* (meaning lord). Barren women were considered a disgrace; a woman's worth was determined by her fertility and how many children she was able to bear. Men were polygamous while women were expected to be monogamous. For women, divorce was no longer an option for any reason. The freedom of the past was a mere memory.

Greece: Misogyny and Boy Love

Ancient Greece, a far different culture from those in the Mideast, is considered to have been one of the most civilized cultures of its time. However, women were still mistreated in this cradle of Western civilization; they were chattel to be owned or used as their men saw fit. The love that most relationships are based on today was unknown and unwelcome; marriage was an economic partnership in favor of the male, and most women went directly from being their father's possession to being their husband's possession.

The marital situation in Greece was far more bleak than our stately image of Grecian culture usually portrays. Married women were cooped up indoors, out of sight of men other than their husbands. The wealthier the couple, the more isolated the woman was. Noblewomen weren't allowed to shop; they had no claim to any of the family fortune; they didn't even own their own children.

Men were considered the perfection of creation, so the ideal love object was a perfectly formed young man or boy barely into the pubescent years. Men married for economic concerns and would commonly visit the local brothel or ogle young boys for sexual gratification. Women were considered second rate, at best.

Adultery among men was acceptable, but among women it was an offense. Divorce was legal, but if a woman chose to divorce her husband, her family most likely wouldn't take her in again. Since she didn't own property and wasn't allowed to incur debt, she had few options besides prostitution, or another marriage if she was lucky.

Men saved their romantic love for young men and the hetaerae—the highborn courtesans. Unlike the typical noblewoman, the hetaera was usually talented in a multitude of arts. Sexually, musically, intellectually, she was considered vastly superior to a housewife. Men could fall in love with these women, but the relationships were doomed by their very economic basis. Hetaerae were far from inexpensive, and few men could afford to keep one for their own personal use and continue to fund their household.

Pederasty was considered completely normal. Romantic love between an older man (the teacher) and a young man (the student) was idealized and placed on a pedestal. However, masculinity was prized, and most fathers did not accept their sons becoming the submissive partner of an older man. A double standard? Yes, much like the man who wants to have sex with his girlfriend but wants to marry a virgin. Once a youth reached a certain age, he was expected to put aside his proclivities and marry. When he was older, he could take a young male lover and continue the cycle.

There is quite a bit of controversy over just how entrenched homosexuality was in Grecian culture, and some schools of thought declare that bisexuality was much more common than homosexuality.

Rome: Adultery As a Pastime

Roman life, though it still subjugated women, required that they be more resilient and active than their Grecian counterparts. A good Roman housewife was expected to run an efficient household while her husband was away on military campaigns, which meant that she must know something about money and business matters.

Divorce laws were changing, too. Though women still could not own property, there were now three forms of marriage, one of which allowed a woman to completely retrieve her dowry from her husband after a divorce. If her father gave her away in *usus*, he retained guardianship over her. Should she be unhappy, she had merely to present a written notice of divorce, pack up her goods, and return to her father's home. Husbands had to work to keep their wives happy; otherwise, they might lose that expensive dowry. Women became more autonomous, avoiding the helpless demeanor prevalent in Greece.

Adultery was illegal in Rome, but was pursued with religious fervor. One of the few sexual acts that was illegal, it carried the risk of discovery; the added thrill of the illicit seemed to create an almost addictive quality. Divorce became common, and marriages were broken up with no more than an announcement of "Take your things away." Childbearing became passé; who wanted to raise children in this type of atmosphere? Abortion and other available forms of contraception were popular among those who could afford them; others practiced infanticide.

To counter the drastic decline in birth rate, which could spell disaster for a country at that time, Augustus Caesar enacted the Julian Laws in 18 B.C.E., the most important one of which was the *Lex Julia de adulteriis*. This law categorized adultery as a federal offense rather than a civil concern—at least for women. By preventing men from killing their adulterous wives (though they were allowed to kill an adulterous daughter) and requiring them to charge a woman in court, these laws instituted adultery as a matter of state importance.

A man was allowed to kill the offending partner in his wife's adultery if he caught the paramour with his wife. He was then expected to dismiss (divorce) his wife and bring her to justice. If he refused to do so, he would be considered an accessory to the crime and would be charged as such. The burden would then fall upon her father. If he, too, failed to bring her to court, then any citizen of the State might charge her and, if a conviction ensued, the accuser would win part of her money. Once convicted, the State confiscated half of her dowry and one-third of her other property, which affected not only the adulterous woman, but her husband. She would then be exiled.

Men faced criminal charges if caught with a married woman, though they retained the freedom to be adulterous with prostitutes as long as they produced heirs with their legitimate wives.

Other Julian laws denied the right of inheritance to bachelors, spinsters, and barren wives. Women who bore three or more children were granted special privileges. Childrearing became popular, and childless men and women were taxed at a much higher rate than parents. Because men outnumbered women, Augustus revoked the restrictions on marriage to freedwomen, and only senators were denied the ability to marry below their status. Children from the resulting marriages were granted legitimacy.

However well intentioned, the vast majority of these laws were failures. The tide had turned on Roman civilization, and there was no shoring up the dissolution that was beginning. The populace refused to rally behind Augustus's authoritarian policies. It could not have helped that Augustus's own daughter, Julia, was well known for her sexual exploits and her disregard of her father's moral strictures.

Forcing her to publicly acknowledge her adulterous nature in court—in accordance with his own laws—Augustus exiled Julia to the island of Pandateria, where she lived under house arrest and was not allowed wine, spirits, comforts, or much company. After a few years, Augustus allowed her to move. She eventually died of tuberculosis. When Julia was sent to Pandateria, Augustus ordered one of her lovers to commit suicide and exiled the rest of them.

Julia had a daughter, also named Julia, and the child continued in the footsteps of her fun-loving parent. Like her mother, Julia II was eventually sent into exile. Before she left, she had taken up with Ovid, the poet, and was ostensibly the cause of his expulsion from Rome. While it is not believed that they were lovers, the story is that he neglected to accuse her of some debauched act that he supposedly witnessed. The more probable reason for his exile is the nature of his writing, his connection to Julia II being an excuse. The sensuous nature of Ovid's poetry was in direct opposition to the emperor's moral strictures.

The Descent into Christianity

As Rome disintegrated, and as the Middle Eastern religions grew more strict, Christianity began to rear its head and ascended with an ascetic vengeance. Virginity became the ideal, and the original meaning of the very word *virgin* was altered. The term referred to a woman who was subjugated to no man, who owned herself. Eventually, it came to mean a woman who had never had sex. Sexual relations between a husband and wife were considered impure, but more desirable than fornication, a term that pretty much covered anything except sex with the goal of procreation. While earlier civilizations had been misogynistic, the very nature of Christianity made them look almost kind in their treatment of women.

Thanks to Genesis, blame for the world's ills was placed squarely on Eve's shoulders. The supposition that she was created from Adam as a helpmeet, rather than an equal partner, paved the foundation upon which modern society bases many of its attitudes toward women. In most other religions in the past, at least women and goddesses weren't assigned an inferior beginning. While not mirrored in the mortal realm, equality did surface for women in many of the divine legends.

In Christian legend, the apostle Paul was one of the main instigators of the concept that woman is the source of evil. He managed to effectively purge any feminine aspects from the Christian religion. With his insistence on the subjugation of women, the superiority of the male, and the evils of sexuality, he forged a branch of Christianity that exists to this day in many of the fundamentalist denominations.

There have been attempts to soften this misogyny in order to encourage a return to Christian ideals. Proponents explain away Paul's scriptures in the Bible as being indicative of the feelings at the time in which they were supposedly written. If this is so, then shouldn't these same scholars, with a view of the modern times in which we now live, reject the literal meaning of these writings? Shouldn't they create a new paradigm for their religion based on updated views of the nature of womankind and feminism today? This doesn't seem to be happening.

The Catholics maintained a reverence for Mary who, though a watered-down version of the goddess Isis, can still be considered a legitimate representative of feminine divinity. While denying women rights over their own bodies, the Catholics have a warm spot in their heart for the mother of Jesus, and they consider her sacred and holy. With the rise of Pauline philosophy, Christianity destroyed the last vestiges of the Goddess that had managed to migrate into the new religion. With this rejection, they obliterated the last remnants of any positive view of feminine sexuality.

Unfortunately, even Mary lost her sexuality. The proposition of "immaculate conception" rejects the idea that human sexuality might have a divine nature; only God would do as a divine lover. Only the denial of mortal flesh could enable Jesus' pilgrims to find their spiritual communion with Mary.

When we examine Jehovah's insistence on absolute obedience, we find the roots of Christianity's rejection of physical passion. When two people develop a strong attraction, their devotion to Jehovah becomes diffused. To ensure unquestioning obedience, there must be no outside factors to influence the pilgrims' emotions and heart—hence, no passionate love. Passion is reserved for devotion to one's god.

Thus, the new religion promoted spiritual communion with deity as the only truly acceptable form of love. The concept of human as divine was disallowed. The divine was separated from nature, above and outside the human experience. Only through unwavering attention to the deity, and the denial of the self as a holy instrument, could mortals aspire to please the new god. By rejecting the body as impure, one relegated all bodily functions to an unclean state. Therefore, sexuality became divorced from the divine.

Perhaps the indulgences of the Roman Empire led to this denial of the flesh, but with the Christian rejection of sexuality, the battle against lust created an obsessive double standard still rampaging through our culture today. By assigning sex the power to tempt and betray, early Christians transformed the nature of lust into a demon. Rigid abstinence almost always creates an obsessive fixation. Many of the early devotees spent their time in masochistic pursuits to subjugate their sexual urge.

Anorexia, abstaining from the pleasure of food and drink, living in uncomfortable surroundings, and the self-infliction of deliberate pain—such as the hair shirts of the monks, flagellation, and beating one's back with spiked boards—all became common attempts to sublimate personal pleasure. Suffering was idealized. This rejection of human pleasure promoted obsession and paranoia. The mere sight of a woman was enough to convince some devotees that the forces of darkness were urging him to sin.

The arrival of St. Augustine during the third century C.E. brought additional strictures against passion within marriage, along with the concept of original sin. Since all births are the result of sexual desire, St. Augustine maintained that simply being born brings a person into sin. He even attempted to present a treatise on how reproduction might have occurred without fornication in the Garden of Eden.

Augustine maintained that: "In Paradise, then, generative seed would have been sown by the husband and the wife would have conceived . . . by deliberate choice and not by uncontrollable lust." He went on to hypothesize that a man could have an erection and ejaculate without an accompanying orgasm, and that the woman could refuse to enjoy intercourse. This concept reduced sex to a bloodless, passionless act solely aimed toward procreation and, therefore, acceptable in the eyes of the Christian God.

Of course, there was no way that Christianity could keep its adherents happy with this state of affairs and, over the years, the religion soon began to slip into its own form of debauchery. Homosexual practices sprang up among the monks, and nuns turned to lesbianism. With no other outlet for their sexual energy, they turned to one another. Those higher in the priesthood often took concubines. Power was abused with the rape of young women in their congregations. By emphasizing that it was the will of God that women should submit to them, these priests found many unwilling partners who were afraid to disobey them.

Gluttony became another substitute for sex, while others sublimated their needs through the rigid control of anorexia. When the Inquisition arose, the sexuality of women took on a supernatural quality and became the scapegoat for just about every ill that the world had ever manifested.

The Burning Times and *The Hammer of the Witches*

In 1484, the Papal Bull of Pope Innocent VIII had officially given the Inquisition in Germany a free rein. With this one document, he turned the power of life and death over to bloodthirsty bounty hunters. Local priests and nobles in some of the more remote parts of Germany didn't want to help the witch hunters in their quest, so the pope decreed that the Inquisition was to receive whatever help it asked for. Anyone who refused to aid the inquisitors could find themselves in danger of becoming a target for the inquisitors.

Pope Innocent handed over power formerly invested in the local authorities to the Inquisition:

> We therefore, desiring, as is our duty, to remove all impediments by which in any way the said inquisitors are hindered in the exercise of their office, and to prevent the taint of heretical pravity and of other like evils from spreading their infection to the ruin of others who are innocent, the zeal of religion especially impelling us, in order that the provinces, cities, dioceses, territories, and places aforesaid in the said parts of upper Germany may not be deprived of the office of inquisition which is their due, do hereby decree, by virtue of our apostolic authority, that it shall be permitted to the said inquisitors in these regions to exercise their office of inquisition and to proceed to the correction, imprisonment, and punishment of the

11

aforesaid persons for their said offences and crimes, in all respects and altogether precisely as if the provinces, cities, territories, places, persons, and offences aforesaid were expressly named in the said letter. And, for the greater sureness, extending the said letter and deputation to the provinces, cities, dioceses, territories, places, persons, and crimes aforesaid, we grant to the said inquisitors that they or either of them joining with them our beloved son Johannes Gremper, cleric of the diocese of Coonstance, master of arts, their present notary, or any other notary public who by them or by either of them shall have been temporarily delegated in the provinces, cities, dioceses, territories, and places aforesaid, may exercise against all persons, of whatsoever condition and rank, the said office of inquisition, correcting, imprisoning, punishing, and chastising, according to their deserts, those persons whom they shall find guilty as aforesaid.

And what crimes were the witches apparently up to? Many of their misdeeds were considered sexual in nature. Not only were witches accused of tempting men and women into carnal acts, they were also accused of causing impotence and sterility, an interesting juxtaposition of charges. Pope Innocent VIII detailed the crimes against God in his Papal Bull *Summisas desiderantes*, (December 5, 1484) as such:

It has indeed lately come to Our ears, not without afflicting Us with bitter sorrow, that in some parts of Northern Germany, as well as in the provinces, townships, territories, districts, and dioceses of Mainz, Cologne, Tréves, Salzburg, and Bremen, many persons of both sexes, unmindful of their own salvation and straying from the Catholic Faith, have abandoned themselves to devils, incubi and succubi, and by their incantations, spells, conjurations, and other accursed charms and crafts, enormities and horrid offences, have slain infants yet in the mother's womb, as also the offspring of cattle, have blasted the produce of the earth, the grapes of the vine, the fruits of the trees, nay, men and women, beasts of burthen, herd-beasts, as well as animals of other kinds, vineyards, orchards, meadows, pasture-land, corn, wheat, and all other cereals; these wretches furthermore afflict and torment men and women, beasts of burthen, herd-beasts, as well as animals of other kinds, with terrible and piteous pains and sore diseases, both internal and external; they hinder men from performing the sexual act and women from conceiving, whence husbands cannot know their wives nor wives receive their husbands; over and above this, they blasphemously renounce that Faith which is theirs by the Sacrament of Baptism, and at the instigation of the Enemy of Mankind they do not shrink from committing and perpetrating the foulest abominations and filthiest excesses to the deadly peril of their own souls, whereby they outrage the Divine Majesty and are a cause of scandal and danger to very many.

The Malleus Maleficarum, or *The Hammer of the Witches*, was written in 1486 by the German inquisitors Heinrich Kramer and James Sprenger. Essentially a guidebook to torture, the *Malleus Maleficarum* evolved from the witch craze that was sweeping Europe. With the book's publication, the debate within the Catholic church over the validity of witchcraft was abruptly put to rest. In no uncertain terms, the *Malleus Maleficarum* stated that witches and witchcraft existed, that witches worshipped Satan, and that torture and death were justifiable means to ending what was seen as a scourge on the face of the earth. The *Malleus Maleficarum* gained the pope's stamp of approval.

Many of those accused and convicted were Gypsies, Jews, homosexuals, and herbalists—people who threatened the power of the Church or who stood outside what by then was the acceptable religious persuasion. Heretics and Pagans convicted by the Inquisition lost their land, and many wealthy landowners abruptly found themselves branded as witches. The Inquisition offered a wonderful opportunity for the Church to enrich its coffers.

The Inquisition's death toll is uncertain. The nine million claimed by modern revisionist historians is far too high to be supported by the birth rate over a 250- to 300-year period; however, it is estimated that several hundred thousand people were killed for crimes against the Church, an incredible number when you consider the low population at that time.

The *Malleus Maleficarum* documents the depths to which the Church had fallen, practicing tortures that were as barbaric and horrendous as any that Hitler's Nazis thought up. Victims' feet and legs were thrust into boots filled with boiling oil, the infamous thumbscrews actually crushed fingers, the rack disjointed bodies, women were raped with everything from a cock to a red-hot iron poker, and being flayed alive was a popular torture. All of these were common methods the inquisitors used to garner confessions. Confession led to death, but an easier death than if one had denied the accusations. There was no escape from the butchers once one accused.

Women's sexuality was now seen, at its very core, as evil. Women were considered a vile contamination used by the devil to taunt men into turning away from God. According to the *Malleus Maleficarum* "A woman is beautiful to look upon, contaminating to the touch . . . a necessary evil . . . an evil of nature . . . a liar by nature . . . since they are feebler both in mind and body, it is not surprising that they should come under the spell of witchcraft . . . a woman is more carnal than a man. . . . All witchcraft comes from carnal lust, which is in women insatiable."

Given the repression of the times, is it any wonder that the Inquisition created a sadistic regime of torture, rape, and murder for its victims? Or that, in an effort to purge and deny their own sexual cravings, these men shifted the blame for their sex drive onto the shoulders of women and gay men and used the witch hunts as a demented form of gratification? Church leaders saw the chance, through confiscation of victims' properties, to enrich their treasury and enlarge their sphere of control. These were dark times, and dangerous ones, for anyone who angered a neighbor who was willing to turn them in to the Inquisition.

Courtly Love

Even as the flames of the stake raged across Europe, courtiers were idealizing women as visions of loveliness to be admired, loved, listened to, but never touched. Courtly love could never be consummated, for when it was, as we see in the legend of King Arthur, the world crumbles and the kingdom falls. Lancelot and Gwynyfyr followed their hearts and destroyed a mythical utopia.

On a side note, I find it interesting that anachronistic groups idealize this time period. The real Camelot is thought to have been an old fortress, and the real Arthur is thought most likely to have been a barbarian king who lived during the sixth century. Historians often credit *Monty Python and the Holy Grail* as being a more accurate representation of the era's grubbiness than such movies as *Excalibur*, yet the whole Arthurian mythos has become a utopian dream for medieval re-creationists.

Back to courtly love. Relationships founded on courtly love were expected to remain platonic. While sex was slowly becoming connected with love, unrequited love was the most romanticized. Here we find the virgin and the whore prejudice. Women were either ladies, never to be subjected to a passion considered base and all-consuming, or they were witches and whores, impure and therefore targets for torture. Unfortunately, that dichotomy exists today—women are "good girls" or "bad girls," while men are simply men.

The Rise of the Puritans

In a surprising twist, we find that during the 1600s and 1700s the early Puritans were actually liberal compared to the Catholic church at the time.

While women still had few rights, sex within the marriage bed was considered acceptable and even desirable. Though publicly condemned, quite a number of people apparently had active adulterous or premarital sex lives.

Contradiction ruled. In an effort to war against the Roman Catholic movement, the Puritan movement viewed celibacy as a sin, a product of the devil's cunning. Marriage became a civil matter rather than a sacred ritual. Martin Luther, the founder of Lutheranism, advocated good food, drink, and making merry for curing temptation. He also promoted sex within marriage as natural and untainted, even though he considered women (as did most men at this time) to be weak, frail, and lacking in intelligence.

Unfortunately, when the Puritans turned away from Roman papal rule, they also turned away from the beginnings of the Renaissance and all that this period of enlightenment brought with it. Sex within marriage might be acceptable, but romance and familiarity were discouraged. Endearments were forbidden; even the use of a husband's or wife's first name was against the Reformation's belief system.

However, the Puritans gave women a step forward in their basic human rights. Divorce became a civil matter, and women could win a divorce and a settlement if they so desired—especially if cruelty had been present in the marriage. Men were discouraged from disparaging their wives in public. Respect for one's partner was encouraged. It was only a century or so later that the zeal of evangelistic beliefs took root in the Puritan movement and spread throughout the members.

And yet . . .

Still the fires and hangings and drownings continued to rage unabated across the European skyline, a swath of hatred against women, homosexuals, Gypsies, and anyone who deviated from the norm. The frenzy spread to Britain and would soon spread to the new colonies of what would later become the United States.

The Restoration: Sex As a Natural Process

One positive result to come out of the Age of Reason was the restoration of sex as a natural urge, divorced (for the most part) from religion. During the 1600s and 1700s, rogues, gallants, and rationalists flourished. Sex became a game, to be approached with a cool demeanor and without emotional frippery. Both men and women, at least among the upper crust, considered romance ridiculous; one lover could easily replace another. Dalliance was favored over commitment.

At the opposite end of the spectrum during this same time, the Puritanical movement began its slide toward the repressive nature with which we generally associated it.

Along with the changes taking place on an emotional and sexual level, society was also changing. Manners became of tantamount importance; the expectation that one would behave in a socially acceptable manner was rigid and unwavering. Women, while freer now to explore their sexual desires, were still relegated to a lesser status and indeed, during this Age of Reason, men threw aside the notion that women were evil and, instead, ascribed to them the inborn nature of irrationality.

Sexuality during Victorian Times

As we emerged into the Victorian era, the era of Romance, sexual divisions somehow got turned around. Women, "good" women, were not only free of the association with divorce and evil, they were considered devoid of sexual desire beyond a kiss and a pat. Men were seen as the animalistic ones, not to be trusted. A woman was never to uncover more of her skin than necessary for fear of setting off a man's violent and passionate nature. She was not to be led astray by the seductive ways of a rogue. This idealistic view of women put them on a pedestal and, once again, stripped away their right to their own sexuality. Chaste love was extolled; only prostitutes were allowed to feel sexual desire. Motherhood was deified; however, one might wonder just how these women became mothers, but logic has never been part and parcel of human existence.

Men couldn't control themselves, and women were responsible for that lack of control, but now it wasn't a deliberate action that caused this state of affairs. The fires that had scorched the soils of Europe were mere embers; the screams had died; the pagans were conquered; the witches and heretics were lost into the flicker of a nightmare. The collective soul of womankind was safe from the devil.

During this period, we find a great schism between the public and private faces of sexual love and lust. A married woman's nightgown from the Victorian era often had a hole near the pubic area, and this was the only way many a husband accessed his wife for intercourse. Women focused on their homes and children, at least, those that had the means. The poorer classes were, as usual, ignored and left to starve and slave away for survival. Men idolized their wives, holding them up as paragons of virtue. The Victorian home was prudish, free from any mention or sign of bodily functions, a peaceful haven from anything that might destroy that sense of serenity and niceness.

It comes as no surprise that women and men couldn't live up to these standards. Sex, while no longer considered sinful, was once again relegated to a base instinct, and all the effort to rise above the carnal caused a backlash.

Modern BDSM (bondage, domination, and sadomasochism) began to make an appearance. While various aspects of BDSM have been around since time began, the Victorians plied it into an art form. Even as budding psychiatrists were labeling all kinkiness as perverse and abnormal, spanking and bondage were present in the brothels and erotic literature. One of the common themes in Victorian erotica is the older man overwhelming, spanking, and then deflowering the innocent nubile teenager.

Corsets, which had been around since the time of the Egyptians, took on a new and renewed life feminizing women—to such an extent that women were not above removing ribs in order to fit into the desired stereotypes that were popular then. However, it is often overlooked that corsets also did the work of a bra and were, to some degree, a helpful undergarment.

The Victorian era gave us prudery, yet it also gave us the beginnings of the modern underground fetish movement. Extremes always coexist, but the two would eventually lead to, at least in the United States, an almost schizophrenic view of sexuality.

The Twentieth Century and Sex: Here We Are

Flappers, bohemians, born-again virgins, nice girls don't, let it all hang out, AIDS, vibrators and manacles, free love, the Pill, sex, drugs, and rock and roll—there's no way to pigeonhole this last, wild century when it comes to sex. In one hundred years, we've gone from ankle-length dresses and keeping our pregnancies secret to watching porn videos with our lover on our VCRs and DVDs. We go to strip clubs, we come out of the closet, we hang up our leather wrist cuffs over our beds in plain sight.

We've got a long way to go before alternative sexuality becomes acceptable in mainstream circles, and there are still many cultures that repress women's and children's rights. Genital mutilation occurs all-too-frequently in some Middle Eastern and African cultures, fundamentalists see evil behind every fig leaf and in every apple, but as a race, we have come a long way from the past millennia of repression and witch burnings.

Which brings us to the rest of this book, and your relationship with your own sexuality. Knowing where we've come from should help you understand what went into creating any lingering guilt trips and shame that you may have regarding your sexual nature. Congratulations—you are the child of five thousand years of debauchery, repression, and sexual prejudice.

We've got a long way to go toward developing a healthy attitude toward sex in our culture, but maybe we can get there together. Are you ready for the journey?

CHAPTER TWO

Sex and Human Nature

sthir_ gang_vartah stanamukular_m_valilat_kal_v_lam
kundam kusuma_aratéj_hutabhujah
ratérlilag_ram kimapi tava n_bhirgirisuté
biladv_ram sidvérgiri_anayan_n_m vijayaté

O mountain-daughter; this cave so deep that it could still
the Ganga's torrents, this fire pit tended by Kama where
Rati dances, this secret cleft which draws the eyes of your
ascetic Lord, from whence this line of hair climbs like a
creeper to bear your heavy breast-buds: Lady, is this your navel?

SAUNDARYALAHARI, 42

Sex—it's everywhere we look, yet for many people, it's nowhere in their lives. Sex causes more problems and more joys than just about any other part of our lives. Wars are fought over sex; sex is used as a weapon, a bribe, a teaser, a promise, a reward, a threat, a sin. Sex is vilified and extolled. There are probably more songs written about sex than about anything else. Movies are saturated with it, books emphasize it, television uses it to sell commodities. Men are expected to be sexual giants; women are expected to be both the virgin and the slut.

So is it any wonder that we are so confused? That we have such double standards? Sex is vital to our natures: it helps our skin and our blood pressure;

it revitalizes relationships; it's fun and a good stress reliever. And yet people titter and clam up about sex. Until very recently, sex wasn't discussed aloud or in mixed company.

We are sexual beings. Children can have orgasms, and many children masturbate regularly unless their parents scare them out of it. Eighty-year-old men can still father children; women in their nineties can still have great sex. We are sexual from the moment we are born until the day we die. Illness can detract from our sexuality; attitude, religious beliefs, and age may slow us down, but we are still sexual creatures.

Great Sex: Attitude Makes a Difference

Imagine two scenarios. In scenario one, a man and a woman (we'll call them Lucy and John) are having sex. John caresses Lucy's breasts; he runs the fingers of one hand along her nipples while he slides his other hand down between her thighs. Lucy winces; she needs more time. She's dry and a little sore as he presses her clitoris too hard. She wants more foreplay. She wants him to kiss her ankles, nibble on her toes, run his tongue along the curve of her back, but she's embarrassed to speak up. She has been told that sex is a natural function so why can't she slide into the groove quickly and easily? Lucy keeps her mouth shut and, in a few minutes, when John enters her, she isn't turned on enough to reach orgasm. She's left high and dry without having climaxed, and she feels cheated.

In scenario two another couple is having sex. We'll call them Jake and Marla. Like John, Jake rushes things a little, focusing on Marla's genitals and breasts but ignoring the rest of her body. But in this case, Marla gently reaches down and takes hold of his hand. Jake pauses, looks at her and asks, "Is something wrong?" "No, sweetie," Marla says. "Nothing's wrong, but I'd love it if you'd kiss my ankles, if you'd run your hands all over my body. You know how that drives me crazy." Jake gets very aroused when Marla expresses her needs and her desire for him to touch her, and he happily spends more time on foreplay. When they finally reach intercourse, their sex is deeper and richer because she's fully in the experience. Her orgasm shakes her to the core, and Jake can feel the ripples of her energy through his own body.

You might say, in the first case, that John was a thoughtless lover, but I propose that Lucy cheated herself out of a better sexual experience because of her reluctance to speak up. Now, true enough, not all men respond well to suggestions and requests, and not all women are comfortable expressing their needs. However, the fact remains that if you want something in your sexual relationship—or any relationship for that matter—you can't expect your partner to be a mind reader. You must ask for what you want, and you must know what you want before you can ask for it.

Now consider two more couples. First we have George and Susan. Susan is a larger woman. She has always been large, and some of her previous partners have made rude comments about her size, but George insists that he finds her sexy and attractive. However, Susan refuses to make love with the lights on, and she constantly apologizes for not being "as pretty as the supermodels." Their sex life is suffering because of her low self-esteem, and Susan resists all of George's encouragement that she wear sexy lingerie and perfume and consider herself sexy. If this pattern keeps up, George may become exasperated and leave, and then Susan will probably chalk it up to the fact that she's a larger woman, refusing to take any of the blame for the relationship's failure.

Now meet William and Tara. William is disabled and in a wheelchair. He has feeling in his lower body, but cannot use his legs. Tara constantly tells him how sexy he is, and he believes it. He sees her look at him with desire and accepts that she means what she says. He dresses well and takes pains with his appearance because it feels good to him to do so. Tara never seems embarrassed by his disability, and when he does need her help, he never feels like she's "doing him a favor." He accepts that he is a brilliant, handsome man and that she's as lucky to have him as he is to have her. He knows how to turn her on, asks her what she wants, and isn't shy about stating his own needs. They have a wonderful marriage, and it will probably last many years due to their mutual respect, not only for one another, but for themselves.

Attitude is the key factor here: attitude toward sex, toward expressing one's needs, and toward yourself. You can't expect to have a good sex life if you

- can't discuss your needs and desires

- are embarrassed by sex to begin with

- base your attempts on inaccurate information

- don't treat yourself with the respect you'd give someone else

Developing a positive attitude toward sex takes time and practice for some people. You need courage to face such a personal and often controversial subject, and you must be honest and direct with yourself and your partner. If you feel unready and unsure, don't despair; there are ways to overcome your hesitancies regarding sexual issues.

Seeing Yourself As a Sexual Being

Both men and women worry about their sexuality.

- Am I normal?

- Do other people want that too?

- Is his penis supposed to curve like that?

- Help! I don't know my way around down there! Where's her clitoris?

- Why do I want sex so much?

- How can I increase my sex drive?

- Is it "wrong" to want him to touch me there?

24

- What would she think if she knew that I wanted her to suck my cock?

- Am I a pervert?

- She's ten years older than I am; how can I be aroused by her?

- He's my father's best friend; how can I want to have sex with him?

- I'm a mother; I'm not supposed to be sexual, am I?

- She's my grandma; how can she still want sex?

Questions such as these run through everybody's thoughts at one time or another. The first key to accepting both yourself and others as sexual beings is to gain knowledge. The more informed you are, the better you'll understand your own body as well as the body of your partner(s). You'll also find that the more you read about the nature of sex and the body, the less reticent you may be about discussing sex and desire. Once you learn to see your body as natural and not something to be ashamed of, you will be more able to talk about your needs and the needs of others.

Female Sexual Anatomy

Most people know that women have a uterus, where a baby will grow if it is conceived, and they know that women have a vagina, where the penis is inserted, but beyond this the wealth of misinformation is astonishing. I knew a man once who thought women peed out of their vaginas. Therefore, I'm going to give you some basic anatomy here. First, from a frontal view; second, the view from between spread legs.

Women have a pair of ovaries, where eggs are produced. Once a month, during ovulation, an egg will erupt from the follicle where it ripened and travel through the fallopian tube into the uterus. (The ovaries generally alternate in producing an egg.) The body will have prepared a lining in the uterus to receive the egg. If no conception takes place, both the lining and the egg disintegrate and are shed during the monthly cycle of menstruation.

The typical menstrual cycle runs between twenty-one and thirty-five days, averaging twenty-eight days. Usually between two and four ounces of blood and fluid are lost during the menstrual cycle. The blood and lining exit the uterus through the cervix, then through the vagina, which extends for a varying number of inches inside the woman.

The vagina is important to a woman's sexual experience. It is lined with a mucous membrane, and reaction to arousal produces lubrication fluid. As sexual arousal heightens, the inner two-thirds of the vagina expands. While the inner vagina is not as sensitive as the clitoris, there is a "G spot" that can trigger erotic arousal. Its placement and existence are debated by doctors, but many women swear they have found it.

When a woman has an orgasm, the walls of the vagina rhythmically contract. Women can learn to exercise their vaginal muscles through Kegel exercises (which are described in chapter 3). The vagina lies near the back part of the labia minora. On either side, small organs called Bartholin's glands produce a secretion during arousal.

On the external side of things, the mons veneris is the rounded, hair-covered cushion of flesh that resides over the pubic bone. The labia majora consist of two folds of fatty tissue that extend from the mons veneris between the legs. Between the labia majora rest the labia minora, which surround the vagina. A woman has three openings in her pelvic area—the vagina, the urethra through which she urinates, and the anus, through which she eliminates waste. Above the urethra, you will see the clitoris and the hood and shaft of the clitoris.

The clitoris can be likened to the penis. It is one of the most sexual spots on a woman's body and by stimulating it alone, with or without intercourse, chances are she will have an orgasm. When a woman is aroused, the clitoris and the labia minora fill with blood, and the clitoris exposes itself outside the hood and shaft. Upon orgasm, the swelling of the labia minora and the clitoris subside.

If a woman is a virgin, she will have a hymen, a membrane that partially covers her vaginal opening. The hymen can be broken by strenuous exercise, so lack of a hymen doesn't mean a woman has had sexual intercourse. This membrane has a small opening that allows menstrual fluid to pass out of the body. This also allows a woman to use tampons during her menstrual cycle whether or not she's ever had sex.

A woman feels sexual arousal all over her body, which can be triggered by touching any number of erogenous zones on her skin—the nipples, the inside of her arms, the back of her ankles, the nape of her neck. Women are capable of multiple orgasms in a single sexual encounter.

If you want to explore your sexual anatomy and develop a working knowledge of what you have and where it is, you might get a hand mirror and take a look at that area, often referred to as *down there.*

Male Sexual Anatomy

When we think of the male's sexual system, we tend to think of penis and balls, and that's all. While the penis is the primary sexual organ for men, quite a few parts make up the male genitalia.

When we look at a naked man's pelvic area, we first see his penis and scrotum. The penis consists of erectile tissue that, when flaccid, is between two and four inches long. When engorged with blood, it becomes erect, and the average penis extends from five to seven inches. If a man has been circumcised, he will no longer have a foreskin extending over the glans or "head" of his penis. If he has not been circumcised, there will be a flap of skin, which is pushed back for cleaning.

The penis rests over the scrotum, the sack-like bag containing a man's testes, or testicles, which produce sperm. There are usually two testicles, but a man who has had testicular cancer or a birth defect may have only one.

27

The penis extends into the man's body. The vas deferens extend from the testicles up through the body and carry the sperm cells to the junction between the prostate and the Cowper's glands—which secretes seminal fluid—and the bladder, which secretes urine. The seminal fluid (or semen) is a fluid that provides a method for the sperm to travel to and in the vagina, and the fluid also provides nourishment for the sperm. In the male, both semen and urine travel through the urethra tube to the opening on the head of the penis. However, it is a physiological impossibility for a man to urinate while he is ejaculating, so you do not have to worry about urine seeping out with semen.

The head of the penis, or the glans, is the most sensitive part on most men, along with the vein that runs down the underside of the shaft of the penis. When a man is aroused, the penis will fill with blood and become erect, thereby readying him for sexual intercourse. Men can learn to orgasm without ejaculating seminal fluid by learning tantric techniques, and can, therefore, learn to have multiple orgasms. This takes practice, however, and overcoming years of stereotyping about the male libido.

Contraception and STDs

Whenever a man and a woman have sex, there is always the possibility of pregnancy unless medical conditions prevent it or proper precautions are taken. The choices for birth control have primarily fallen on the woman's shoulders. However, with the advent of HIV and AIDS, condoms should be routinely included in every sexual encounter between a nonmonogamous couple, whether you know the other person's sexual history or not.

In fact, I'm going to go so far as to say that until you know each other so well that you would put your life in the other person's hands, and unless you are in a committed, monogamous relationship, you should be using a condom along with any other contraception you may choose. It doesn't matter whether you are a heterosexual couple or a same-sex couple—condoms are the only safer sex alternative we have.

Sex can be deadly if you contract AIDS. The world is held captive by this epidemic, and the simple fact is: when you have sex with a person, you are in essence having sex with all of their previous partners as well. You cannot tell what diseases a person might have by how they look or how nice they are. I don't want to hear that you trust the Goddess to watch over you; don't be a fool and don't tempt fate. The gods help those who help themselves. Fate doesn't play favorites.

Unplanned pregnancy is bad enough on both your psyche and the environment, but do you really need to play Russian roulette with your life? If you are a woman, remember: the pill won't protect you from STDs. Neither will a diaphragm, a sponge, or an IUD. A condom and some spermicides containing nonoxynol-9 are the only effective barriers to the HIV virus, and they are not always foolproof. If you are a man, don't believe the rumors. Yes, you *can* contract HIV from a woman, and yes, you *can* spread it whether you have symptoms or not.

In addition to AIDS, there are other serious STDs out there just waiting for the stubborn and the uninformed.

- Syphilis can be cured easily; however, if left untreated this disease can cause a host of problems, including death.

- Gonorrhea, also easily cured, can lead to sterility and damage to the reproductive organs, as can chlamydia.

- Herpes, the same base virus from which we get cold sores and canker sores, has no cure and is easily transmitted between partners. While it doesn't lead to death, it's an ongoing health problem for those suffering from it.

- HPV (human papillomavirus) manifests in several ways, for example genital warts and cervical dysplasia, and if not treated promptly, can lead to increased risks of cervical cancer.

- Hepatitis C has no known cure and can lead to chronic hepatitis and an increased chance of liver cancer. This disease can be passed sexually as well as in other ways.

- HIV/AIDS, of course, is a complex syndrome that generally leads to death and, at this point, has no known cure.

So why am I writing about being sex-positive and then hitting you with this information? Because most people don't take STDs seriously, and there are some dangerous and lethal time bombs out there. I want you to read the next paragraph and memorize it, commit it to heart, and make it a part of your personal ethical system; there's no excuse for any other type of behavior.

> If you are old enough to have sex, you are old enough to take responsibility for your own health and for ensuring that you don't endanger someone else's health. If you are old enough to have sex, you are old enough to learn how to prevent unwanted pregnancy and to handle the mistakes when they do happen.

Don't blind yourself to a new partner's potential ability to lie or sneak around on the sly. Protect yourself. Insist on condoms.

Slang Terms: Talk Dirty to Me, Baby

"But what do I call 'it'?" Let's face it, people are uncomfortable talking about sex. Part of that discomfort comes from the belief that sexual terminology is "dirty." But when we sterilize it, anatomical terms like *vagina*, *penis*, and *clitoris*, sound too clinical. And euphemisms like "down there" and "weenie" sound childish and silly. Well, the truth of the matter is that terms like "cock" and "fuck" have been around for hundreds of years and were used without shame until the modern era. Once we reclaim them from the gutter, we can use them without sounding like we're aiming for a career in a porn movie, working toward a medical degree, or making up "baby" talk. Some common and not-so-common slang terms (and you will see these in this book, so deal with it and smile) include:

- vagina: pussy, cunt, slit, yoni (a Sanskrit term), honey pot, hole, lotus, the celestial garden, bush, beaver, snatch, tail

- clitoris: clit, hornet, pearl, lotus bud, cum button, twat

- buttocks: ass, backside, buns, butt

- breasts: boobs, tits, melons, gazongas, headlights, knockers, hooters

- penis: dick, cock, rod, shaft, prick, peter, dong, John Henry, lingam (a Sanskrit term), the jade scepter, Johnson

- testicles: balls, nuts, family jewels, rocks

- semen: cum, ejaculate, jizz, jizzum

- orgasm: come, shoot a wad, climax, get your rocks off, get off

- arousal: turn-on, a hard-on, wet, horny, hot and bothered

- fellatio: giving head, sucking cock, giving a blow job, going down on, sucking off

- cunnilingus: eating out, eating pussy, going down on, licking, giving a tongue bath, muff diving

- masturbation: playing with self, jerking off, jacking off, twiddling yourself, fucking yourself, spanking the monkey, choking the chicken, hand job

- sexual intercourse: fucking, screwing, making love, balling, going all the way, getting laid, doing her/him, having sex, sleeping with, having vanilla sex (sexual intercourse without kink), doing it

- anal intercourse: cornhole, going around the world, Greek sex, going to Greece, fucking in the ass

You may not be comfortable with all these terms, but you should attempt to find a measure of comfort with some of them so you have a working vocabulary for discussing sexual issues. If we can't speak about sex in all its variations, how can we expect to come to a mutual understanding with our sexual partners about what we want and how we want it?

Spend some time at this. Begin by reading the various terms until you can look at them without blushing. Then, when you are alone, try saying each word aloud, as if you were reading off a vocabulary sheet. Then practice using each word in a sentence until you find the terms that you are most comfortable with. Remember, your goal is not to use these words as gutter language, but as part of your vocabulary so you aren't resorting to vague euphemisms and childish nicknames that disempower the nature of your sexuality.

Private Exercise: Getting to Know Your Body

It is vital to get to know and become comfortable with your body. Begin when you have some time alone, when you aren't going to be interrupted. Try to give yourself at least an hour or more. If privacy is a problem, tell your family that you are going to take a bath, and then lock the bathroom door. In fact, even if you have the house to yourself, a relaxing bath or shower can be a great prelude to this exercise.

If your bathroom doesn't have a low-light setting, consider using a touch light or light several candles (making sure they are not near anything flammable and are secure in their holders). Sprinkle some bath salts or bubble bath in the tub. You might want to play some music like Gabrielle Roth's *Ritual*. Fill the tub with warm water and undress slowly. Allow your hands to graze your body as you remove your shirt, your pants or skirt, and your undergarments. Do not judge your body; simply feel the skin under your hands.

Run your hands lightly over your body—over your torso, your chest or breasts, your penis or pubic mound, your legs. Slide your fingers up your arms; caress your shoulders gently. Don't aim for arousal. Simply get used to the feel of your skin under your fingertips. Is your skin smooth? Do you have scars? If you have tattoos, does that skin feel different than the unmarked skin? Simply observe.

When your bath is ready, step into the tub. (If you do not have a bathtub, then take a leisurely shower with bath gels or scented soaps.) Let the water surround you. Focus on the feeling of the water touching your flesh. How do you connect with the water? What does it feel like against your naked body?

Stand in the tub; feel your feet and ankles surrounded by water as your body is surrounded by air. Feel the difference between the elements as they caress your body. Now either sink into the tub or step into the spray, and immerse yourself in the sensations of water on your skin. Roll your neck gently from side to side, then flex your shoulders. Take a deep breath and exhale slowly. Let the water work through the tension in your muscles. Reach up and stretch, then sink into the sensation of the water again.

Take a handful of lather and slide it over your skin. Enjoy the slipperiness as your hand slips across your naked flesh. Do not judge, do not fret, merely focus on the soap as it coats your body. Take a cup and dip it in the water, then pour thin streams of water over different areas of yourself, from different heights. The water will cool if you pour from a greater distance. What does this feel like compared to the warmth of the waves surrounding the rest of you? Or if you are in a shower, adjust the pulse of the droplets— bend over and let the spray play on your lower back, then turn and face the showerhead and imagine yourself under a waterfall. Play, enjoy, and explore your spirit through exploring your body.

When the water begins to cool, step out of the tub and wrap yourself in a robe or towel. Blow out the candles or take them into your bedroom. If you have no other place for privacy, arrange a cushion of towels on the bathroom floor.

Thoroughly pat yourself dry. Use a thick towel and press it to your skin. When you are dry, stand naked and enjoy the play of air on your body. How does it feel to be clean, fresh out of a bath, naked as the day you were born? Focus on the sensation of being nude and free of clothes and jewelry.

Play some hypnotic, trance-inducing music, and keep the room warm enough for you to stand naked comfortably. Using a lotion or oil in your favorite scent, begin to lightly stroke your body. Rub gently, with a circular motion, as you cover your body with the fragrant unguent. Direct your attention to whatever body part you are touching at the moment, and follow the feeling as your fingers cover the surface of your skin. You may find yourself aroused sexually, or you might find this relaxes you, and you are becoming sleepy or entering a light trance.

If you have a disability, then adjust the instructions as necessary for your particular situation. Unless you are totally disabled, you can still move parts of your body. With whatever ability you do have, begin to follow the beat of the music with your body, whether it be with your arms, your shoulders and head, or your whole body.

Begin a slow, rhythmic dance as you slide your hands along your flesh, letting your feet follow the cadence of the music. Breathe evenly, slowly, and deeply. Let your hands tell the story of the music to the rest of your body. Let them become the drummer, the singer, the pianist. If you find yourself wanting to sing along or make noise, then do so. This is your time to dance with yourself, to use motion and touch to explore the nature of your body and to love yourself while doing so.

Feel the curve of your belly, and love the curve of your belly.

Feel the silken skin of your chest, and love the silken skin of your chest.

Feel the strength of your thighs, and love the strength of your thighs.

Cup your breasts, and love the pendulous mounds of feminine flesh.

Grasp your cock, and love the shaft of your masculinity.

Use the music's slow rhythm and your own deep breathing to allow yourself to slide into a trance as you delve deeper into the mysteries that surround your body. If you end up masturbating, no problem, but that's not your goal. You are making friends with your body, getting to know it— curve and hollow, bulge and mound, smooth skin and rough flesh. You are not to criticize, but simply to observe, greet, claim, and move on.

If you find your attention repeatedly starting to wander, you may be tired and should continue the next day. Or ask yourself if you're trying to avoid this intimate contact with yourself? If the latter is true, then you must determine why you are afraid of getting to know your body. After all, it is the temple of your soul and should be revered and loved and pampered the way you would any sacred land or object. When you can claim your body as your own, you will feel at home in it and be more comfortable with someone else's touch.

Overcoming Embarrassment: Now That I Am Comfortable with Me, How Do I Approach My Partner?

One of the best ways to approach sexual difficulties or desires with your partner(s) is to discuss the issues. "But how can I overcome my embarrassment in talking about sex with other people?" you ask.

This is where honesty is vital and good communications skills are absolutely essential. If you don't know how to communicate well, especially when dealing with potentially inflammatory issues, then you won't be able to discuss your sexual issues with your partner. To begin, you must first assess whether or not your partner is open to communication about sex. If he or she blocks you and will not talk about these issues, there are three common reasons for this behavior.

One: Your partner may be just as embarrassed to talk about sex as you are, in which case you can sit down together and discuss the embarrassment as an issue in itself. Treat it like an obstacle you can work together to overcome. If you both want to free yourselves from this block, then unite and agree that you will not let an outside factor such as shame or repression defeat your relationship. Often, the very act of admitting that communication is a problem will free it up some. The relief of confessing one's feelings will sometimes trigger a release.

Two: Your partner's upbringing may have instilled a great deal of shame or guilt about sex and created a discomfort in discussing it. This is a harder block to overcome, and though you might be able to approach the subject and overcome the problem alone, if the difficulty and shame are severe, you may need to visit a couples counselor together. If lack of communication forms a wedge between you and you encounter continued resistance to discussion, then you should make your worry clear and insist on finding someone who can help. Always research a counselor or therapist before setting an appointment, however, and make sure you both feel comfortable with the professional you've selected.

Three: At times your partner may be afraid of hurting your feelings. He or she may also sense a lack in the relationship but doesn't want to make you feel inadequate. You should prepare yourself for hearing complaints or desires that might make you uncomfortable. You might not be the only person in the marriage or relationship that desires change or the ability to openly discuss sexual issues.

Let me give you an example, a personal one, of the latter situation. My husband, Samwise, and I have been together since 1992. When we met, we both made a mistake that could have ended our marriage. While sex was wonderful, it wasn't totally "swing from the chandeliers" time for me, but it was far better than my previous relationship. I *assumed* that Sam's quietness signified a deep and thoughtful nature, and that it would be only a matter of time before he became more assertive in bed.

Meanwhile, he *assumed* that because I was now in a "stable" relationship, I would quiet down a little and not be as adventurous as he knew I had been in the recent past. Neither one of us discussed either of these assumptions. In 1998, we began to have problems in the bedroom. Sex became shallow and boring to me. Sam was happy with our sex life, though he could sense something was wrong.

I was afraid to talk to him. I wanted something that I wasn't sure he could give or would be willing to give. I wanted him to tie me up and blindfold me, so I could experience the sensations on a more intense level. I also wanted to practice sacred sex, but it didn't seem a priority for him. What neither he nor I recognized was that when someone possesses a strong personality (like me), that person sometimes needs a place in their life where they can release control, where they can experience being vulnerable.

A friend of mine had recently gotten into BDSM, and she told me about a book she was reading called *Different Loving: The World of Sexual Dominance and Submission*. I pulled away because I recognized myself in her description of the book. I didn't want to experience pain, but I wanted those restraints, and I didn't want to be the one doing the restraining. However, I also knew that Sam had a real aversion to BDSM. How could I suddenly turn to him and say, "Honey, would you kiss me there, and there. Oh, and while you're at it, would you tie my arms up and chain me to hooks over our bed?"

Eventually, our problems became more pronounced. He joked to cover it up, and that really turned me off. He was skilled as a lover, there was no problem there, and he did his best to please me the way he thought I wanted it. But it wasn't working for me. One day I finally broke down in tears and told him that I wanted him to be stronger, to quit making stupid jokes while we were having sex. I wanted to be tied up. He shook his head. No, he couldn't tie me up. We argued and ended up looking at each other with new understanding, saying, "How in the hell did we ever manage to stay married this long?" and "What do we do now?"

It is important to note that nothing was resolved that morning, or for several months to come. We had sex, and I went through the motions. He quit being goofy in the bedroom, and it helped a little. But our relationship was still strained. Then one day he agreed to try what I had asked. I was overjoyed. But the minute he started tying up my wrists, he stopped and said, "I can't do this." And we were back to square one.

A few days later he initiated the discussion again. We talked. He expressed his fears that he would be hurting me. I pointed out that I wasn't asking him to hit me, to whip me, or to do anything else that might hurt— all I wanted were those restraints on my wrists. I also reminded him that he knew he would stop if I asked him to.

The next time we had sex, he tied me up with a silk scarf. When he saw how much it turned me on, he was convinced that it would be okay. Samwise has no interest in being tied up and doesn't understand why it turns me on, but he does find my own excitement arousing. So on those occasions when I need the wrist cuffs or velvet cord, he's more than willing to wrap them around my wrists and lovingly knot me into bondage.

While I will discuss what I, and many other people, get out of bondage in another chapter, I bring this up here because it is a good example of how open and honest communication can save a marriage or relationship. It is also a good example of how it can take more than one session of talking; we had to analyze and compromise and find ways to meet my desires while not forcing him into a position that made him uncomfortable. Our discussions hurt both of us. No one wants to admit that there are sexual problems in a relationship; no one wants to admit that they aren't meeting their partner's needs and that maybe, just maybe, they won't be able to meet them.

If Sam had not been willing to work with me, to overcome some of his fear, I don't know if we'd have much of a relationship today. If I had not been willing to let go of some of my fantasies, I doubt if our marriage would have lasted.

As it is, our relationship is much stronger because of the steps we took. The experimentation with bondage led to experimentation with various sex toys, which was a realm that *I* was uncomfortable with at first. Turnabout time. Sam wanted me to be comfortable masturbating.

In a previous relationship, my partner had turned away from me time and again in favor of his own hand. To me, my partner masturbating pretty much meant that I wasn't "woman enough" for him. And if I had masturbated, it would have given my ex the excuse he needed to avoid sex totally.

I knew that Sam still masturbated at times, and while I tried not to let it bother me and it didn't interfere with our sex life, I was uncomfortable with it. And when he asked me how I masturbated, I couldn't talk about it.

Finally I decided that I didn't want to be uncomfortable with any part of my sexuality, so we bought a selection of vibrators, and I learned to pleasure myself. For the first time in my life as an adult in a committed relationship, I brought myself to orgasm. I liked that feeling of empowerment. I also discovered that quite often my orgasms while masturbating took me into a realm that sex itself, tied up or not, didn't seem to offer.

Here came the dragon of intensity. I wanted to experience what I was feeling alone, with Samwise. Around that time, I also knew that I wanted to write this book, but how could I write about sex, magic, and mysticism if we couldn't blend the three together in our own experience? So I laid it out for him. I wanted to write a book about sex and the divine; would he be willing to go into hours of in-depth research in the bedroom with me? Would he agree to let me talk about our own sexual problems and practices so I could help others who might be in similar situations? I didn't have to ask twice. Samwise has given me full permission to talk about our sex life in these pages.

So I thumbed through my books, including the ones I had bought on Western tantra. I went to the bookstore and watched the gleam in the clerk's eye as he totaled up my sex-book shopping spree. I ordered so many books on kink and alternative sex through an online bookstore that, every time I logged into their site after that, their recommendations were of the sort that probably made the clerks think I was a Class-A Pervert. I began to read, and then we began to develop our own sexercises.

Our sex life and our relationship is better than it's ever been. We've developed a deep connection, unspoken but acknowledged. And he's very proud of my career, whether it be writing about sex or writing one of my mysteries.

When something works, we discuss it and remember it for the next time. When something doesn't work, we talk about it and either adjust or discard it. But we adhere to the following basic rules of communications etiquette.

- Always use "I" statements. "I feel that I'm not understanding you" as opposed to "You never make yourself clear." This allows you to claim a feeling of discomfort without placing all the responsibility for it onto your partner's shoulders. This helps you share the burden of the situation.

- Watch your body language. Are you saying you'll be open to something while crossing your arms, indicating that you're actually closed to the idea? Your body's reactions to a touchy discussion can tell you more about yourself than you may realize.

- If you've had communication problems with your partner for a long time, or if the issue is a significant one, it will probably take more than one attempt to talk it through to a resolution. Agree at the start of the discussion that you will not expect miracles to occur regarding an issue that may have taken years to build up.

- ❧ Remember that some sexual problems, including the lack of a sex drive, can have a medical basis. At times, fatigue and burnout can cause problems, and you may have to address how you prioritize your time and schedule. If you cannot pinpoint a reason for the lack of sexual interest, you should schedule an exam with your physician.

- ❧ Don't discuss sexual problems while in the bedroom. Granted Samwise and I did just that, but we should have taken them to a neutral room where the energy of the situation might have been a bit more diffused.

- ❧ Be willing to compromise. "You tie me up, and I will give you oral sex in return."

- ❧ Prepare yourself ahead of time for potential resistance and anger. Nobody wants to feel inadequate as a lover, and your partner, when confronted with a problem, may take it badly or be so embarrassed (especially if they thought your relationship was satisfactory) that they become hurt and angry. This is one reason why "I" statements are so important—they diffuse the sense of blame.

- ❧ Use precise language. If you say, "I'm not getting turned on enough before you enter me," your partner isn't going to know that you actually mean, "I'd like you to give me oral sex." Be sure to couch requests or desires in a nondemanding manner.

- ❧ Assess your sex life, indeed your relationship, regularly. Make it a weekly or monthly activity. It may seem rather analytical, but is your connection with your partner any less important than the bills? Many people have budget meetings to discuss their financial status, why not a sex analysis meeting?

- If you think the situation is going to be rather volatile, agree ahead of time to a stated time length for the discussion. Stick to that time frame, and before you end the session, agree on the next time that you will sit down together to continue. You might want to agree on a second time before you begin, so you feel free to speak without fearing that your partner will shut out the idea of another discussion.

- Respect your partner's desires, no matter how strange they may seem. You don't have to agree to participate in them, but recognize that this may be important to your mate. If you poke fun of or demean their fantasy or humiliate them, you are hurting someone you love, and you may do irreparable damage to the relationship. If Samwise had told me I was nuts for wanting bondage, rather than just stating that he found it distressing, I would have been embarrassed and unable to bring it up again. I might have gone looking for someone who would take me seriously.

- If your partner is adamant about not wanting to discuss sex, or if there is no sense of compromise in sight, it may be time to consult a therapist or marriage counselor. You can only do so much, and one person cannot carry the entire responsibility for a relationship. It may seem embarrassing, but many couples seek therapy to shore up the sagging points of their marriage or partnership. Therapy isn't an automatic stamp marking you as prime for divorce or a breakup.

After the Discussion: What Next?

Once you and your partner have come to a better understanding of each other's needs, you may find that you have similar sexual desires. If this is the case, then there should be no problem proceeding unless one of you discovers later that you really don't want what you thought you wanted and the other one loves it. If you both want to experiment with sex magic, sacred sex, or BDSM, then you should research your chosen pursuit and practice, as always, safe, sane, and consensual sex.

But what if, for example, one of you wants to experiment with bondage and the other one doesn't? How do you compromise? How do you cope with this? Well, you could do what Samwise and I did: talk and talk, unearth the objections, and see whether there are any misconceptions leading to those objections.

If you are both clear about the issue, and one of you still says "no," then you should explore whether something else will substitute that you can both agree on. Perhaps one of you isn't comfortable with tying the other one up; you might be comfortable blindfolding your partner. Or maybe you don't want to swallow semen during fellatio, but you are willing to suck his cock until just before he climaxes. Whatever the compromise, both parties have to feel that they are getting something out of the experience.

When you first attempt a new position, activity, or pursuit, it may be awkward so try it more than once. Don't write off an experience as useless or boring until you have developed a bit of adeptness and know for sure that it's not the newness or uncertainty of what you are doing that is leaving you cold.

On the other hand, if you absolutely hate your experiment, there's no reason why you should continue, unless you are simply afraid to step outside of your comfort zone. This is an important distinction. When we fear new experiences, we can easily mistake that sense of fear for distaste. It's much easier to stick with the familiar, rather than work at something new. So be honest with yourself. Did you really dislike the taste of her pussy, or are you just concerned that you don't know how to go down on her right? If you are worried about performance, ask how you're doing. Ask for suggestions. You shouldn't be expected to be a mind reader.

Have fun with your experimentation. When something strikes you as silly; examine why you find the situation funny. Sometimes sex is ridiculous, and if we saw ourselves in a porn flick we'd probably crack up laughing. Once we remove ourselves from the situation for a while, we might decide that what we were doing is most definitely a turn-on.

This goes for masturbation, too. Don't be afraid to try new things, think up new fantasies. There's no reason you can't go out and rent a porn flick for yourself. There's no rule saying that you can't eye that cucumber on the counter with salacious thoughts. You don't have to tell anyone what you did. In fact, I'm a big fan of keeping fantasies private—that way you won't be labeled a pervert, and telling people what you fantasize can take the oomph out of the fantasy. Having a secret about yourself can make you feel a little mysterious and sexy.

Don't be ashamed of what you do. As long as you aren't hurting anybody—including yourself—whatever you're doing is normal for you. Be proud of your sexuality.

I've Got a Problem: My Partner Simply Refuses to Experiment

In every instance where another person is involved in your sex life, you must prepare yourself for the possibility that your partner might resist your ideas. What will you do if they simply refuse to participate in any experimental sexual behavior? You have several options. You can

- ☙ confine your desires to fantasy and use them during masturbation. This may be enough; only you can make that decision.

- ☙ suggest a marriage counselor and hope that your partner is willing to join you. You must, however, prepare for the inevitability that the therapist will tell your partner, "You don't have to do this if you don't want to." It's vital to remember that no person has the right to force their desires on anyone else—whether it be husband, wife, friend, or stranger. If your partner is truly distressed about what you want from them, you can't expect them to participate happily. You have the right to ask that they consider it, but not the right to insist that they go through with it.

꾜 find a different partner for your experiments. In this case, you must have your long-term partner's approval, and you must consider the consequences of your actions before carrying them out. If you agree to an open marriage of equality, it works both ways. How will you feel when your partner has sex with another person? How will they feel when they know you've been out with somebody else?

꾜 dissolve your relationship and hope to find someone with whom you are more sexually compatible. If there isn't much holding you together, this might be your best choice. If you both love each other, then maybe you need to reconsider how important the desired sexual activity is compared to what you would lose by saying good-bye. Remember: Often what we are seeking is within, not without.

Sometimes nothing will make a relationship work. The sex life is often the first area to suffer in a failing partnership or marriage, and though you can try to rescue it, sometimes it's best to admit defeat and move on before it gets worse. Only you and your partner will know when that time comes. If you blind yourself to problems in the relationship, you may find yourself sitting there alone one day after having refused to listen to your partner's complaints.

It's My Partner Who Wants to Experiment, Not Me!

Oh gods—first your partner starts reading all these sex books, then he or she complains to you about your sex life. What are you supposed to do now?

- ☙ "What do I do? She wants me to use her vibrator on her, and I don't know if I can do that! I don't know *how* to do that."

- ☙ "He wants to have sex in a public place where we might get caught. I'm afraid of getting in trouble."

- ☙ "She says our sex life isn't spiritual enough. She's been reading all these books on tantric lovemaking, and now she wants me to make love for two hours instead of twenty minutes! How can I possibly do that?"

- ☙ "My husband just handed me a copy of *Different Loving* and pointed to the part on submission. He says he wants to lick my toes and be my sex slave. I think I'm repulsed, but I'm not sure."

Let's turn the tables for a moment and imagine that your partner comes to you with a request that you either don't know how to fulfill or you find repugnant. What should you do? Before you give them a knee-jerk reaction and shout, "No, you pervert!" stop and consider their request.

Are you simply afraid that you don't know the proper techniques and will look like a fool or won't be able to fulfill their needs? If this is the case, then confide your fears and ask that you both study the subject together and work on it slowly so you have time to accustom yourself to the new activity. Any new sexual technique needs time for exploration and adaptation to your own use. Neither partner can expect themselves or the other person to be an adept on the first try.

Does the experiment sound risky, perhaps unsafe? Examine the components of what your partner wants and see whether you can work around the parts that might entail potential danger. Use Velcro wrist cuffs rather than tight ropes if you fear cutting off circulation. Buy a flail that leaves no marks on the body and stings lightly rather than a riding crop that might slash and cut if used improperly. Or take a class (yes, there are classes in proper BDSM techniques) from a qualified professional so you know the ins and outs of what you are attempting.

Do you find the proposed activity silly, and you're afraid you'll embarrass your partner by laughing? Find a compromise. If you know that you'll crack up when he walks in with his cock covered in whipped cream like a banana split, then suggest that you apply Kama Sutra edible oil instead. A cock covered with cinnamon-flavored lubricant can be quite wonderful and erotic, without having to think of your boyfriend's genitals as a giant ice-cream cone.

Are you embarrassed by your lover's idea? Ask yourself where your embarrassment stems from, and see whether there's a way you can work through it.

If you find the suggested activity too far beyond your comfort zone, then maybe you can start small. If you can't masturbate in front of him, can you lightly caress your breasts and body as you apply lotion all over? This is one way to become comfortable touching yourself in front of someone, as well as being good for the skin. After you are comfortable with this, perhaps you can move on to focusing on the genitals.

Do you simply find the desired experiment repulsive? If she wants you to urinate on her (commonly called golden showers) and you find the concept repugnant, then you must stand up for your rights and say, "No, I can't do this." If you offer a compromise and she's unwilling to accept it, then you must be prepared for the possibility that she will leave or find someone else to play with in this manner. Never compromise your own sense of dignity for someone else, though—whether they threaten to leave or not. Self-esteem takes a long time to build up and a lot of work to nurture.

What If I Truly Think That I Am (or My Partner Is) Abnormal?

Wanting to fuck your dog isn't the wisest choice, for you or the dog, but I assure you, there are people who fantasize about this and some who've actually done it. While it's definitely not in the norm, it isn't something for which you can or should be committed, though I state clearly here that it borders on animal cruelty, and you should never engage an animal in a sexual act because they can't protest.

If you *only* want to have sex with your German shepherd, then it's time to consult a therapist. And if you hurt your animal during these acts, *immediately* seek help for both yourself and your pet.

By the same token, if you find yourself desiring to have sex with a minor or a child, *seek therapy immediately*. Inappropriate behavior with a youngster can destroy their life. The numbers of molestation abuse show that this activity is not confined to a minority of society. It's a very real and prevalent threat to all children. Sexual predators abound. Far too often, they try to find justification for their actions. The fact remains: While children are sexual with themselves at a young age, they should not be engaged in sexual activity. They aren't prepared for it, and it can and will scar them in ways that most people can't comprehend.

Sadomasochism is not in and of itself wrong, but when forced upon an unwilling partner or when it's carried to extremes within a consensual relationship, there's a definite problem. If you have doubts about how far is too far, then you need to sit back and seriously assess what it is you're doing and why you're doing it.

Many Pagans partake in polyamory or panfidelity. However, when you ignore rules about safe sex and dismiss your partner's feelings of jealousy or inadequacy without care or thought, you may be jeopardizing your relationship and you need to address it.

Be conscious about your sexual choices. Examine your prejudices to see where they stem from so you can make informed decisions rather than knee-jerk reactions. And if something just feels wrong to you, then listen to your intuition and avoid the activity. Sexuality is to be enjoyed, not tolerated.

CHAPTER THREE

Masturbation, the Kundalini, and Magic

> I sing the Body electric . . .
> The man's body is sacred, and the woman's body is sacred;
> No matter who it is, it is sacred.
>
> WALT WHITMAN, "I Sing the Body Electric"

Perhaps one of the most sensitive issues we face when talking about sexuality is masturbation. Speaking openly about masturbation always sets off a rash of giggles, blushes, or, worse, stony silences or reprimands. Masturbation seems to be more taboo in most circles than homosexuality. Is this any wonder when we examine the childhood strictures heard from our parents and other authority figures?

- "Don't touch yourself *down there*."

- "Get your hands out from under those covers!"

- "Self-abuse will make you blind (grow hair on your palms, and so on)."

- "A woman who uses a vibrator won't be able to enjoy intercourse with a man."

- "Masturbation is a juvenile pursuit, no one in a mature sexual relationship needs to masturbate."
- "Only men masturbate; women don't need it."
- "Masturbation is a sin!"
- "Good boys don't."
- "Nice girls don't."

We all recognize some of these phrases. Most likely, at some point during your childhood, someone scolded you for touching yourself. People simply don't want to admit that children can enjoy sexual feelings from the time they are babies. It shakes up the Judeo-Christian paradigm that we live with. However, research shows that young children can have orgasms and, given freedom, most children will masturbate.

Our resistance to this knowledge may stem from a fear that people will try to rationalize pedophilia if we accept children as sexual beings. Unfortunately, some perverts do adopt this mindset, causing terrible harm. The existence of monsters like this prevents us from safely helping children learn how to appreciate and love their bodies. No rational person in our society will agree that it's okay for an adult to take advantage of or hurt a child in this manner. Anyone promoting pedophilia has more than a few screws loose—people know right from wrong, they can act in appropriate manners and take responsibility for their actions. When they don't, we have to prevent them from harming others.

Religion also plays a role in the masturbation issue. Good boys and girls don't touch themselves because masturbation is a sin. Unfortunately, much of what is pleasurable in life is a sin in many belief systems, as we saw in chapter 1. The concepts that life equals suffering and that open sexuality is sinful are not limited to the Judeo-Christian religions, as we have discovered. However, since most of us stem from a Judeo-Christian culture, we carry around guilt from our past, conveniently tucked away in our memories. Sometimes we don't even know that we are packing this baggage.

Opposition to open discussion of masturbation and to acceptance of it as a normal human behavior was illustrated in the outcry following former Surgeon General M. Jocelyn Elder's suggestion that masturbation should be taught in schools as a form of safe sex. Dr. Elders was railroaded from her position; she left office in December 1994. The furor over what was a remarkably good suggestion amazes me; yet, considering the prudish nature of our society, it's not surprising that Dr. Elders was put to the rack for her comments. We have one of the most amazing double standards on sexuality of any westernized country. Sex is extolled and vilified at the same time.

The truth of the matter is that to fully enjoy sexuality, to connect with our bodies in the most intimate way, we must be able to give pleasure to ourselves. When we have no partner, or when our sex drives are disparate from our partner's, masturbation provides a much-needed release. And if we are interested in sex magic, but have no partner—well, guess what? We're going to have to be comfortable masturbating to experience the connection with the divine that tantric forces can bring to us.

Women and Attitudes toward Masturbation

Men and women approach masturbation differently. Current statistics show that 90 percent of men masturbate, and about 60 percent of women do. However, since women tend to be shy about admitting the truth on this subject, it's hard to gauge the validity of statistical studies on this issue. Men are generally freer in talking about masturbation, while women tend to be more embarrassed. There are several reasons for this.

For one thing, we women don't see our genitals like men do. We don't touch our urethra like a man holds his penis during urination. Women don't see dramatic effects of arousal like a man does when he gets an erection. Men are more familiar with the physical aspects of their sexuality.

The closest some women ever get to touching themselves is when they insert a tampon (if they even do that). Since the majority of women have children, and baby making is a messy business that requires an incredible focus on the body as it changes, especially the reproductive area, it's amazing that we're still embarrassed over our cunts and clits and breasts. Men in our society are encouraged to express their sexual selves far more than women. When we talk about our periods or sex, a lot of women refer to their genitals as "down there" and many men refer to both women's menstrual cycles and any sexual dysfunction as "female problems."

Unless there's some medical reason to prevent it, women bleed every month for approximately forty years. Women can create life in their bodies. Why can't women enjoy their sexuality and talk about it like adults? Shame and guilt are two of the most insidious power stealers in this culture.

Masturbation and Me: A Personal Story

I admit that it took me a long time to learn to masturbate as an adult and to accept it as something that was not only normal, but also desirable. Why? As I stated in the last chapter, I believed that when I had a long-term partner, I shouldn't need to masturbate. And if he wanted to masturbate, it meant I wasn't sexually desirable. So, although I had masturbated during my teen years, I quit when I hooked up with my ex.

Then I found out that not only were he and I incompatible, but also he had some sort of sexual hang-up and never wanted to have sex. He substituted masturbation for sex, and he withheld sex when he was angry. He used to say, "Why don't you just masturbate?" But I knew that if I did and he found out, he'd have another excuse to avoid me in bed.

This is still not an easy issue for me to discuss. This is personal information, but I am willing to use myself as an example because I know many people have psychological blocks to enjoying their bodies and are too ashamed and embarrassed to talk to anyone about it. I want those of you who feel this way to know that, yes, it is difficult to face, but you are not alone.

When I met Samwise, the sex was good. However, I still couldn't allow myself to masturbate. He asked me why, and I told him. He reassured me that he would be happy if I were to pleasure myself. As I listened to my friends talk about their experiences, I began to feel stunted. Truthfully, I felt stupid. Then, shortly before I realized I needed to write this book, something clicked. I wanted to face my fears and hang-ups.

And so I hesitantly put one foot in the arena. I bought a set of vibrators and began my forays into the world of self-pleasuring. I soon discovered some of the positive side effects. Then, while writing this book, I faced the ultimate in learning to be comfortable with masturbation. I decided to get over my embarrassment about masturbating in front of Samwise. Though I'm still not that comfortable with him watching, I overcame my fear and learned a lot about how accepting he is and how turned on a man can get watching a woman pleasure herself.

So even if you are coming from a background with a lot of sexual hang-ups, a lot of unresolved issues, you can learn to love your body, to pleasure yourself, and to discover your solitary connection to the divine through sex magic and masturbation.

The Place of the Flowers—Communion with the Divine

I am lying in bed; the sun is glimmering through the window. I'm aroused, nipples erect. The sound of the vibrator is almost like white noise, allowing me to ignore the cars on the streets, the crying cats.

The tension in my body builds; I ache with desire, so much that it feels like I'll never be satisfied. Yet I can sense that the edge is near. I let myself plateau, let the energy rest for a moment. In the quiet drone of morning, I feel every pore of my body; every muscle is alive, every cell vibrant. I begin again, take a deep breath, and slowly exhale.

And then, just as I begin to think that I'm not going to climax; then the shift happens. I am on the edge and over, soaring upward, dizzying height sending me reeling, spiraling through the void of the universe to the place of the flowers, where I drift. The scent of roses intoxicates me. I can feel a soft rain of petals. Shadows of a garden surround me as I rest gently in the arms of cloud silk.

I expand out—touch the core of the universe, that primal energy, and they are both there, masculine and feminine. This energy sparkles with the divine. The Blue God; Shiva is dancing. Shakti races through me with her fire as the gentle touch of flowers cushions my descent.

Then I am back to myself, in my bed, breathing softly. Radiant and glowing, I wish that I could live forever in the place of the flowers.

I have no other name to describe this state of awareness. Indeed, I wonder whether this is simply my body's own metaphor for communing with the divine. But names aside, this is a place I've been to several times, and each time the sensation is the same, so I'm wondering just what I may have stumbled onto here. I've searched through old tantric texts for references to "the place of the flowers" and haven't discovered it yet, but I continue my studies. In terms of experiencing this state through sexual intercourse rather than just masturbation, I've had it happen a few times. The first time I had this experience was years ago, when Samwise and I were first together. The last few times came through our experimentation with westernized tantric techniques, especially when we've invoked Shiva and Shakti into our magical rites. The only controls I seem to have so far for reaching this state are

- focusing on Shiva and Shakti during my approach, whether during sex with Samwise or during masturbation

- using the "plateau" method that I discuss later on in "Women: Pleasuring the Sacred Lotus"

So I'm still learning, still experimenting. But each time I reach this state of awareness, I know that it signals a much vaster possibility than I've tapped into yet.

The Basics of Masturbation

Self-pleasuring doesn't necessarily come naturally. Even when you do get rid of the guilt, there may be the problem of "what do I do?" More women suffer from this paralysis than men do, so I will focus more on women during the following sections, but much of the advice can be applied to men as well.

For women, one of the most complete guides I've found is a book called *For Yourself: The Fulfillment of Female Sexuality* by Lonnie Barbach. This little book goes into incredible depth in an attempt to help women overcome their sexual fears and guilt. I will be presenting exercises and suggestions to help you learn to touch yourself without embarrassment. If you are seriously conflicted about these issues, you might wish to start with Barbach's book.

If you are in a permanent relationship, you should decide whether or not to talk to your partner about this issue. I generally advocate honesty in a relationship, but if you truly feel that your partner will be threatened by your need to better understand your body and won't be able to work it out, you may decide to keep quiet about your self-pleasuring.

If you do talk to your partner, be clear that masturbation will not replace your sex life with him or her. There is ample evidence, and I have learned this about myself, that the more a woman masturbates, the more she both desires and enjoys her partner. So self-pleasuring can increase a woman's sex drive. And the more that men have sex and masturbate, the longer they may be able to maintain an erection during intercourse.

Being in Your Body

Many women don't want to think about their bodies. They're so insecure about their looks and so unfamiliar with their own body signals that they ignore a number of both subtle and blatant arousal sensations. I'm not saying that we can or should go around continually feeling stimulated, but if you pay attention to your body, you may find yourself aroused far more often than you expect.

When you walk out into the cool breeze, do your nipples harden? If not, next time focus on the sensation of the wind on your body. When you feel your nipples stiffening, bring your attention to the way your bra or shirt rubs them. Very subtle, but a definite turn-on. Next time you watch a movie that you find erotic, instead of focusing on the plot, let your mind drift to the sensations running through your body. Note what it is in the movie that excites you. Some people find certain types of men or women stimulating. Music is also an aphrodisiac. Remember the *Cheers* episode where Ted Dansen was trying to discover which song turned on Kirstie Alley? (It was The Righteous Brothers singing "You've Lost That Lovin' Feeling.") Fragrances can be turn-ons, or the way a certain texture feels in your hands.

We all have our own personal triggers. For me, music really trips my trigger. I also love the smell of leather and spice, the feel of satin and velvet, and the visuals in certain movies and shows. Being watched can be another turn-on—eyes intensely focused on you. If you can identify what is specifically erotic to you, then you will have an easier time fantasizing and be able to add those triggers to your sex life with your partner.

When you get to know your body and become attuned to your physical state, whether it be horny, tired, energized, or hungry, you will be able to react appropriately to your needs. Are you hungry instead of tired? Do you really want sex instead of food? Listen to your body and pay attention to its signals. If you are too tired for sex, but you really need a long bath, then take one and don't worry about it. If you are aroused, but your partner isn't in the mood, go masturbate instead of wolfing down a chocolate fix. Who knows, they might find themselves ready and willing once they realize what you're doing.

We experienced getting in touch with our bodies in the last chapter, and will be doing more of those types of exercises in the chapters on becoming the Sacred Harlot and the Stag King. Here, we focus on technique and skill.

Kegel Exercises

Kegel exercises are listed in just about every book on sex that has been written since the 1950s, and with good reason: they work for both men and women. What are they? They are simple strengthening exercises to tone the pubococcygeal (PC) muscles that you can do anywhere—at work, at home, in the bathroom, in bed. They don't take long, they won't make you break into a sweat, and no one but you and your partner will be the wiser.

In the 1950s, Dr. Arnold Kegel developed an exercise to help women suffering from postpartum weakening of the PC muscles. Weakening of this muscle often results in incontinence, and now we know that this weakness can aggravate loss of some sexual sensation. Dr. Kegel did not expect to hear that his exercises would help women's sex lives become more satisfying and their orgasms stronger. When he began receiving this unexpected feedback, Dr. Kegel made the connection that the PC muscles are used in sexual intercourse, and since they contract during orgasm, the exercises were, in effect, giving the area a workout.

The best way to locate this muscle, for both men and women, is during urination. When you start and stop the flow of urine, you are using your PC muscle. Begin to exercise this muscle by using it when you're peeing, starting and stopping the flow several times so you can isolate the muscle. After you are comfortable with this, you can begin to do Kegel exercises whenever you like. Simply contract the muscle, then relax.

Start with brief contractions, then add longer ones until you can hold the contraction for a count of four. Begin with a set of twenty Kegel exercises, twice a day. Combine a mixture of long and short contractions until you are performing one hundred repetitions twice a day. This will significantly help to strengthen your sexual PC muscle and should add to both the intensity and the frequency of your orgasms.

Women who want can insert a dildo or finger into their vagina to practice "grabbing" onto a cock. This heightens sensation for men, and it's fun to watch their reactions as well as enjoying it yourself.

Women: Pleasuring the Sacred Lotus

Masturbation is different for everyone. Here, as in all my exercises, don't ignore the rest of your body in favor of your genital area. Start with a slow bath in a warm soapy tub of bubbles. If you have never masturbated before, or you have guilt about it, a bath is a good place to begin. Everyone bathes, and we're used to touching ourselves when we wash our bodies. This adds a sense of safety and comfort to the process.

When you are relaxed, go into your bedroom and shut the door. Make sure you will not be interrupted. It can weaken your future comfort level if someone walks in on you unexpectedly. If you like, wear a sheer nightgown or other piece of lingerie that makes you feel sensuous and sexy.

Light a few candles, put on some music, perhaps light a stick of incense. Let your hands begin to slide over your body. Now begin to focus on your erogenous areas. Gradually, bring your attention to focus on your breasts and nipples. Stroke, pinch, twist—whatever feels good. You can use a scented oil (or unscented if you prefer) to enhance the feel of your fingertips on your skin.

Trail your fingers down through your pubic hair and slide them onto your clitoris. Rub gently, press harder, tickle, tease. Whatever you do, take your time! It takes women longer to orgasm than men. You don't want to feel like you're hurrying things, nor to feel awkward about however long it takes.

Note which areas are most sensitive, what pressure you like, how it feels to slide your fingers inside your vagina. If you have sex toys, now is the time to bring them out. Try out different types of vibrators and dildos. You can use several at once, if you like. You might want to insert a dildo into your vagina while stimulating your clitoris with a vibrating egg. Or use ben wa balls while using a vibrator on your clitoris. Some women also enjoy touching and stroking their anus.

As you become aroused, start picking up the pace of your strokes. Don't forget to breathe. Deep breathing enhances sexual experiences of all kinds. Also, don't be shy about expressing yourself verbally. Let yourself moan, cry out, even speak if you like. Here is where fantasy can come into play, too. Let your imagination run away with you. Nobody ever has to know what you are thinking, or who you are thinking of. If you find it helps to fantasize about fucking your best friend, going down on your next door neighbor's husband, tying up your son's gym teacher, getting it on with the three surfer dudes next door, or eating out your local Miss Dairy Maid, go ahead and do it. Fantasy is fantasy, and you shouldn't feel guilty over what plays out in your head.

When you near orgasm, let yourself rest for a moment. Plateau and take a few deep breaths. Don't wait too long, just long enough to even out at this new level of arousal, then begin again. If you plateau and rest several times, your orgasm will be much stronger. When you are first learning to masturbate, don't plateau more than once or twice, or you may lose your rhythm. As you continue to practice, you will be able to plateau several times, and each time you will reach a new level of heightened sexual tension.

Think of the plateau method as walking up a steep staircase. If you go straight for the top, you will tire and only be able to climb partway. If you take an occasional break, you will maintain your progress and be able to climb higher than if you had not rested. When you get to the top, the view

61

will be much more spectacular than from further below. This is integral to my ability to reach the place of the flowers that I spoke of earlier.

When you reach orgasm, rather than just experiencing it and letting it pass, savor it. You will find, with practice, that you can linger at the peak for longer periods of time if you are used to having orgasms regularly. The more sex you have, whether it be masturbation or with a partner, the better sex will be and the more you will want it. Remember, it may take several tries to be comfortable enough to orgasm. Don't give up!

Men: Stroking the Jade Scepter

Men don't seem to have as many hang-ups, on the whole, as women do regarding masturbation. As I said before, men are used to touching their genitals. I'm not suggesting that men are never embarrassed over the practice or that they're guilt free sexually. Uncontrollable erections, wet dreams, and nocturnal emissions during adolescence can cause worry, guilt, and fear for boys who don't understand that these responses are normal. The view that men are animalistic and women are pure has certainly done as much harm to men's egos as it has to women's sexuality. So men may have to overcome some emotional and psychological barriers to masturbate without shame.

If you like, take a long bath like I recommended for women. Some men like bubbles just as much as women do. When you are done, close yourself in your bedroom. Because men ejaculate during orgasm unless they are practicing advanced tantric techniques, you may wish to take a towel or washcloth with you. You'll want some oil or lotion. Play whatever music you like, and light a few candles.

Begin by caressing your entire body. Most men focus on their cock and balls while ignoring other areas that may be highly erogenous. Take time to explore your nipples, your ankles, your legs and arms. Run your hands over your stomach and buttocks. Fear of homosexual associations may cause some men to be very nervous about touching their anus or their butt, and this is sad. Enjoying the feeling of hands on your ass doesn't mean you're gay. And if you are gay and hiding it from yourself, then you need to do some long and serious thinking about why you're afraid of your true nature.

Use the oil to massage your body as you slowly work your way toward your genital area. Warm a small dab of oil in your hands and lubricate your penis. By now, you are most likely becoming aroused, if you don't have a full-fledged hard-on already. Use fantasy to enhance your experience. It's a safe and healthy outlet and there's no harm in it. Fucking your best friend's wife, going down on the new neighbor who just moved in, being in the center of an orgy of women, even doing the meter reader man—in fantasy, anything is possible.

Grab your cock firmly, and slide your hand up and down the shaft. If you are circumcised, ring the head with your hands and squeeze gently, putting pressure on the underside of the glans. Experiment with different strokes. What feels good to you? Do you want a faster pace? Slower?

Don't rush your experience. Cup your balls in your hand and squeeze. Explore your perineal area (between your scrotum and your anus). The perineum covers the prostate gland, and if you regularly apply pressure onto this area, you will find your arousal stronger. If you have difficulties with premature ejaculation and there are no medical issues causing your problem, you can practice bringing yourself near orgasm, resting for a moment as you catch your breath, then starting again. This start-and-stop technique, my plateau method, has helped a number of men.

Masters and Johnson developed another technique that works. When you are about to ejaculate, grasp the head of your penis where the glans meets the shaft and squeeze for about thirty seconds. You may find your erection subsides a little. Then resume your sex play and build up again. You might also want to experiment with cock rings, which can sustain an erection, and vaginal sheaths during your self-pleasuring.

Some men enjoy the feeling of a vibrator pressed against their penis, and there are toys specifically made to simulate a vaginal sheath—artificial pussy, so to speak. You can order these by mail if you're too embarrassed to go into a sex shop.

When you have reached the point of climax, let yourself slide into orgasm and experience it with your whole body. Don't feel you have to remain silent. Moan, speak, cry out. Sex should be a total experience.

The Kundalini Force

The Kundalini force, the life force of our bodies and spirits, lies coiled at the base of our spine, in our base chakra. There are seven major chakras that lie along our bodies, running up the spine and front of the torso. The first element of this system of energy, or power points, is the base chakra, which rests at our tailbone and leads up to the crown chakra on the top of our head. It is through these points that we run energy during sex magic, meditation, or spiritually focused exercises. The Kundalini tends to remain dormant until awakened.

The Kundalini is most often visualized as a serpent, embodying our life energy, passion, and creativity. By gradually arousing the serpent within and bringing it up our spine, we expand our consciousness and achieve a communion with the divine.

If you awaken the Kundalini too fast, you may find yourself in trouble. The intensity of the forces can be overwhelming and can create some spectacular effects. I found, when waking my Kundalini, that my sex drive went crazy. It's never gone back to "normal" and remains extremely high. Combined with my age (women peak in their sexual desires during their mid-thirties to mid-forties, and I'm smack in the middle of that range), this has been quite a journey. Sometimes I feel like a nympho; every man around catches my eye, and I get horny when someone so much as looks at me. But it's not a bad thing, for a wakened Kundalini also recharges creative and magical energies.

However, as I explain in *Crafting the Body Divine:* You cannot awaken the Kundalini in one area of your life—be it sex or be it exercise—and not have it affect the rest of your life. Be aware; this is not just a lark or parlor game. You are dealing with the primal life force here, the fires of Shiva and Shakti, and it can and will affect you. Passion is one thing, divine passion another.

Once you have begun to awaken the Kundalini, though, you must not try to shove it back down the spine, to repress it. You must work through the energies that it rouses and learn to integrate them into your life. There's no turning back from opening the psyche in this manner. Repression can make you sick—emotionally, physically, and spiritually. Pace yourself according to your own needs, and rest when you need to.

The Nature of Our Chakras

If you were to look at your etheric or astral body, you would see seven points of light emanating from the front and the back of your body. Each point is a swirling vortex of color and, when functioning properly, should be turning in a clockwise direction. Various systems offer different explanations for what energy/functions each chakra controls, but most have more similarities than divergences. If you're interested, read *The Psychic Healing Book*, by Amy Wallace and Bill Henkin. Here, I use some of the more basic definitions and correspondences.

Near your tailbone, right above over your pubic area, you will find the chakra that governs your instincts for survival. This chakra also controls physical energy, and if your hip bones are out of alignment, they can disrupt the flow of energy from the coccygeal chakra up through the spine and thus disrupt the flow of sexual and psychic energy. I found this out when I finally got my hips aligned after a fall I had in 1994. Four years of being out of joint had really blocked my energy channels, and when they snapped back into alignment, I almost fainted from the rush of energy. The first chakra usually runs a bright and vivid red.

The second chakra, your sacral chakra, is found over the womb or penile area, approximately four inches or so below the belly button. The sacral chakra controls your sexual impulses and your sexual-spiritual connections with others. This chakra is the pleasure chakra and usually runs a bright orange.

We move up to the solar plexus for the third chakra. The energy we feel here is what people refer to as a "gut" reaction. The solar plexus connects us with the universe and is also focused on our personal health and emotional well-being. This is the place of harmony between our bodies and our psyches, and it is through this chakra that we sometimes find other energies trying to access our psychic abilities and attention, which is why I suggest checking it every now and then for "cords" from people to whom we do not wish to be feeding energy. The third chakra is located midway between the heart and the belly button and, when clear and healthy, will run a clear lemon or golden yellow.

When we come to our hearts, we find the fourth chakra. The heart chakra reigns over our connections with nature, our families, friends, and everyone we interact with, be they four legged, winged, or bipedal. The heart chakra is the seat of our emotions—our tears, our joys, and our bliss. Here we find the love we feel for a husband, a wife, a child, a mother, a lover, a pet. The heart chakra runs a clear green when it's healthy and in harmony with our natures.

The fifth chakra, or throat chakra, controls our communications with others—both in giving and receiving responses. This chakra also controls our ability to take care of ourselves and take responsibility for our lives. The fifth chakra is located at the base of the throat and runs a clear blue when healthy and functioning properly.

We move up to the center of the forehead and the sixth chakra, which is commonly referred to as our "third eye." Our third eye is our link to a greater perception of the way our reality works, to seeing the connections between concepts and ideas. This is our psychic center, as well, where we process our intuition and hunches. The third eye usually runs a deep indigo.

Lastly, look to the top of your head for the crown chakra. This chakra integrates all parts of our being. It is the gateway to reaching out to the universe and discovering our place within that vast expanse that is both macrocosm and microcosm. It is the doorway through which we enter the body at birth and exit the body at death, or during sessions of astral projection. The crown chakra is a pure, translucent, and brilliant light.

Seven-Step Visualization to Awakening the Kundalini

Take your time with this exercise; you should not rush it. You might wish to complete the seven steps over a seven-week period, or even a seven-month period if you are feeling hesitant about your abilities in this area. Once you start, however, you should complete the cycle. As I said, you can't go back once you start to waken the Kundalini, and you should try to go forward at a pace that is comfortable.

You don't need to memorize the following visualization, though you should memorize the steps and its basic nature. If you like, you can have a friend guide you by reading it to you, or you can tape record it, but for the most part, you want to get the basics down in your mind and go from there.

For each of the seven steps, start out with the following:

▶ Find a comfortable place with no distractions.

▶ Play some music like Gabrielle Roth or Suvarna or Dead Can Dance if it will help you slide into trance.

▶ Stretch out your body, perhaps with some light yoga or simple stretches.

⤖ Settle into a comfortable position.

⤖ Take three deep breaths and close your eyes. Relax and flow into the energy around you.

⤖ Visualize yourself floating against a background of the night and stars (or daylight and clouds if that works better for you). See yourself nude, arms outstretched against the vast expanse of space.

⤖ Reach out with your mind and touch the energy that is flowing through the universe around you—the energy that permeates everything and everyone. Feel the sparks play off your body, off your mind. Revel in the endless nature of the universe that you are an integral part of.

⤖ Examine your etheric body and see the chakras swirling with energy.

Awakening the Kundalini: Step One

Focus on your first chakra, near your tailbone. This chakra is your lifeline to physical life: it helps you remember to breathe; it gives you the adrenaline to move quickly in danger; it alerts you to pain. Examine the chakra carefully. Is it bright red and swirling clockwise? If not, you will want to clear it.

Imagine a bright and sparkling ruby in your hand. Place the ruby against your first chakra and feel it slip into the vortex in your body. Once inside, the ruby begins to burrow through your chakra, clearing out old gunk and debris. See memories of old wounds and physical pains turn to dust and sweep out of your chakra on a sparkling crimson wind.

Imagine your chakra beginning to whirl in a clockwise motion, slowly at first, then faster and faster as the ruby cleans it out. The color flickers and turns into a clear, bright red, and you can feel yourself letting go of old connections that are outdated and useless in your life now.

Now, at the base of your tailbone see a coiled serpent—your Kundalini as it rests, asleep. The energy from the ruby shoots in a brilliant line and falls upon the sleeping serpent's face. One eye slowly opens, and then the other. The snake raises its head, and you can sense that it needs to stretch.

Watch as it raises up, slowly stretching its sinuous body as it flickers its tongue in and out of its mouth. It tastes the energy of your first chakra and very slowly begins to climb toward the vortex, searching, awakening sensations you never knew you had.

When it reaches your first chakra, you find yourself awash in the sensation of being alive—of being in tune with your body, with those reactions that keep you alive. Feel your breath, moving slowly in and out as your lungs bring in air to circulate through your system. Feel the blood pumping in your body, racing through your veins, carrying nutrients and oxygen to every part of yourself.

Take a moment to examine how it feels to be physically alive at this point, to really and truly connect with your body on a survival basis.

Now relax and remove your focus from the serpent. You know it will take some time before the snake makes it to the next chakra, so you let it proceed at its own pace as you relax. Do not attempt to return the Kundalini serpent into a sleeping state; now that it is awake, you must not attempt to repress its growth.

Take three deep breaths, and open your eyes when you are ready.

During the next week or month, focus on your body and its needs. Listen to what it is telling you about your health. Pay attention to your physical self and revel in being alive and part of this wonderful world.

Awakening the Kundalini: Step Two

Focus on your second chakra, midway between your belly button and your tailbone. This chakra is your lifeline to your sexual energy; it helps you to channel your feelings of passion and personal energy. Examine this chakra carefully. Is it glowing orange and swirling clockwise? If not, you will want to clear it.

Imagine a bright and sparkling jacinth in your hand. Place the jacinth against your second chakra and feel it slip into the vortex in your body. Once inside, the jacinth begins to burrow through your chakra, clearing out old gunk and debris. See memories of sexual mishaps, rejections, and hurts turn to dust and sweep out of your chakra on a sparkling golden wind.

Imagine your chakra beginning to whirl in a clockwise motion, slowly at first, then faster and faster as the jacinth cleans it out. The color flickers and turns into a clear, bright orange and you can feel yourself letting go of old relationships and self-conscious feelings that are outdated and useless in your life now.

Now, see a coiled serpent resting in your first chakra; your Kundalini is waiting for your signal. The energy from the jacinth shoots in a brilliant line and falls upon the serpent's face. One eye slowly opens, and then the other. The snake raises its head, and you can sense that it needs to stretch.

Watch as it raises up, slowly stretching its sinuous body as it flickers its tongue in and out of its mouth. It tastes the energy of your second chakra and very slowly begins to climb toward the vortex, searching, awakening sensations you never knew you had.

When it reaches your second chakra, you find yourself awash in the sensation of being sensuous, sexual—feeling the rhythms of your desire, those reactions which bring you pleasure. You can feel your breath, rising and falling, speeding up with excitement. You can feel the heat of your body growing as you become aroused.

Take a moment to examine how it feels to be sexually aware of yourself at this point, to really and truly connect with your sexuality and know that it is awake and aware.

Now relax and remove your focus from the serpent. You know it will take some time before the snake makes it to the next chakra, so you let it proceed at its own pace as you relax. Do not attempt to return the

Kundalini serpent into a sleeping state; now that it is awake, you must not attempt to repress its growth.

Take three deep breaths, and open your eyes when you are ready.

During the next week or month, focus on your sexuality and its needs. Listen to what your body is telling you about your desires. Pamper yourself, indulge in sensuous lotions, oils, and perfumes. Pay attention to taste, touch, smell, sight, and hearing and how they affect your sexual desires.

Awakening the Kundalini: Step Three

Focus on your third chakra, midway between your belly button and your heart. The solar plexus is your lifeline to your gut reactions to people, places, and events. It helps you to channel your feelings of belonging and of harmony with your surroundings. Examine the chakra carefully. Is it glowing yellow and swirling clockwise? If not, you will want to clear it.

Imagine a bright and sparkling citrine in your hand. Place the citrine against your third chakra and feel it slip into the vortex in your body. Once inside, the citrine begins to burrow through your chakra, clearing out old gunk and debris. See memories of misplaced trust, of unheeded intuition, and the results of that neglect turn to dust and sweep out of your chakra on a sparkling topaz wind.

Imagine your chakra beginning to whirl in a clockwise motion, slowly at first, then faster and faster as the citrine cleans it out. The color flickers and turns into a clear, bright yellow, and you can feel yourself letting go of old uncertainties and feelings of isolation that are outdated and useless in your life now.

Now, see resting a coiled serpent in your second chakra; your Kundalini is waiting for your signal. The energy from the citrine shoots in a brilliant line and falls upon the serpent's face. One eye slowly opens, and then the other. The snake raises its head and you can sense that it needs to stretch.

Watch as it raises up, slowly stretching its sinuous body as it flickers its tongue in and out of its mouth. It tastes the energy of your third chakra and very slowly begins to climb toward the vortex, searching, awakening sensations you never knew you had.

When it reaches your solar plexus, you find yourself awash in the sensation of being aware of your place in this world, of being confident and sure of yourself. You hear your inner guidance, and you can see how the patterns of your life work.

Take a moment to examine how it feels to be aware and confident of yourself at this point, to really and truly connect with yourself and know that you are capable and alert.

Now relax and remove your focus from the serpent. You know it will take some time before the snake makes it to the next chakra, so you let it proceed at its own pace as you relax. Do not attempt to return the Kundalini serpent into a sleeping state; now that it is awake, you must not attempt to repress its growth.

Take three deep breaths, and open your eyes when you are ready.

During the next week or month, focus on your gut reactions to people, events, and situations. Listen to what your inner guidance is telling you about the world and people around you. Pay attention to the part of yourself that can see further than your conscious mind, that watches out for you.

Awakening the Kundalini: Step Four

Focus on your fourth chakra, resting over your heart. This is your center of emotion and connection with your loved ones, your pets, your friends, and family. The heart chakra helps you to channel your feelings of love and nurturing. Examine the chakra carefully. Is it glowing green and swirling clockwise? If not, you will want to clear it.

Imagine a bright and sparkling emerald in your hand. Place the emerald against your fourth chakra and feel it slip into the vortex in your body. Once inside, the emerald begins to burrow through your chakra, clearing out old gunk and debris. See painful memories of betrayed love, broken friendships, and loved ones lost to death and the ravages of time turn to dust and sweep out of your chakra on a sparkling peridot wind.

Imagine your chakra beginning to whirl in a clockwise motion, slowly at first, then faster and faster as the emerald cleans it out. The color flickers and turns into a clear, bright green, and you can feel yourself letting go of old feelings of loss and pain, of loneliness and anger that are outdated and useless in your life now.

Now, see a coiled serpent resting in your third chakra; your Kundalini is waiting for your signal. The energy from the emerald shoots in a brilliant line and falls upon the serpent's face. One eye slowly opens, and then the other. The snake raises its head, and you can sense that it needs to stretch.

Watch as it raises up, slowly stretching its sinuous body as it flickers its tongue in and out of its mouth. It tastes the energy of your fourth chakra and very slowly begins to climb toward the vortex, searching, awakening sensations you never knew you had.

When it reaches your heart, you find yourself awash in the sensation of love, for all with whom share your heart. You see the love that friends offer to you, that your family and loved ones give to you, and you are suddenly aware of what a great gift their love is. You sense, in turn, the love that you offer to others, and what a valuable gift it is.

Take a moment to examine how it feels to be filled with love, of all kinds, and to really and truly experience your sense of emotional connection with others.

Now relax and remove your focus from the serpent. You know it will take some time before the snake makes it to the next chakra, so you let it proceed at its own pace as you relax. Do not attempt to return the Kundalini serpent into a sleeping state; now that it is awake, you must not attempt to repress its growth.

Take three deep breaths, and open your eyes when you are ready.

During the next week or month, focus on your heart and your emotions. Do you need to express your feelings to anyone that you are close to? Have you been neglecting people you love? Do you feel neglected by those who are part of your life, and do you need to express your needs to them? Pay attention to your emotional health and your feelings of connection with this wonderful world.

Awakening the Kundalini: Step Five

Focus on your fifth chakra, resting at the base of your throat. This is your center of communication and responsibility. The throat chakra helps you to communicate effectively and to accept responsibility for your actions and your own life. Examine the chakra carefully. Is it glowing blue and swirling clockwise? If not, you will want to clear it.

Imagine a bright and sparkling sapphire in your hand. Place the sapphire against your fifth chakra and feel it slip into the vortex in your body. Once inside, the sapphire begins to burrow through your chakra, clearing out old gunk and debris. See memories of miscommunications and the chaos they caused and of duties shirked out of an unwillingness to take responsibility turn to dust and sweep out of your chakra on a sparkling azure wind.

Imagine your chakra beginning to whirl in a clockwise motion, slowly at first, then faster and faster as the sapphire cleans it out. The color flickers and turns into a clear, bright blue, and you can feel yourself letting go of old incoherent feelings and muddled thoughts. You can feel yourself releasing fears of taking charge of your life.

Now, see a coiled serpent resting in your fourth chakra; your Kundalini is waiting for your signal. The energy from the sapphire shoots in a brilliant line and falls upon the serpent's face. One eye slowly opens, and then the other. The snake raises its head, and you can sense that it needs to stretch.

Watch as it raises up, slowly stretching its sinuous body as it flickers its tongue in and out of its mouth. It tastes the energy of your fifth chakra and very slowly begins to climb toward the vortex, searching, awakening sensations you never knew you had.

When it reaches your throat, you find yourself awash in a flood of words that need to be said, of ideas that must be communicated. You understand that taking charge of your own life is an empowerment rather than a chore.

Take a moment to examine how it feels to be filled with clarity and understanding, with the ability to communicate your thoughts and ideas to others and to accept the driving force for your own life.

Now relax and remove your focus from the serpent. You know it will take some time before the snake makes it to the next chakra, so you let it proceed at its own pace as you relax. Do not attempt to return the Kundalini serpent into a sleeping state; now that it is awake, you must not attempt to repress its growth.

Take three deep breaths, and open your eyes when you are ready.

During the next week or month, focus on your ability to communicate, and try to focus your thoughts so your words and actions are clear. Heed your body language and make sure you aren't giving mixed messages. Look for those places in your life that you tend to give power over to others, and reclaim that energy to choose and decide for yourself. Pay attention to language and the joy of interaction with others.

Awakening the Kundalini: Step Six

Focus on your sixth chakra, resting against your forehead. The third eye is your center for psychic understanding and mental acuity. The sixth chakra helps you to discover the hidden motives in others' actions and words, as well as the underlying factors in situations and issues in your life. It gives you that sense of intuition that comes like a bell ringing out of a silent sky. Examine the chakra carefully. Is it glowing indigo and swirling clockwise? If not, you will want to clear it.

Imagine a bright and sparkling black onyx in your hand. Place the onyx against your sixth chakra and feel it slip into the vortex in your body. Once inside, the onyx begins to burrow through your chakra, clearing out old gunk and debris. See memories of old mistakes based on incomplete information, of misread motives and situations, of hunches ignored, turn to dust and sweep out of your chakra on a sparkling obsidian wind.

Imagine your chakra beginning to whirl in a clockwise motion, slowly at first, then faster and faster as the onyx cleans it out. The color flickers and turns into a clear, bright indigo, and you can feel yourself letting go of old feelings of regret and uncertainty.

Now, see a coiled serpent resting in your fifth chakra; your Kundalini is waiting for your signal. The energy from the onyx shoots in a brilliant line and falls upon the serpent's face. One eye slowly opens, and then the other. The snake raises its head, and you can sense that it needs to stretch.

Watch as it raises up, slowly stretching out its sinuous body as it flickers its tongue in and out of its mouth. It tastes the energy of your sixth chakra and very slowly begins to climb toward the vortex, searching, awakening sensations you never knew you had.

When it reaches your third eye, you find yourself awash in a flood of insights and intuition, of guidance and clear sight. You understand that you are seeing beneath the surface, below the superficial niceties of life.

Take a moment to examine how it feels to be filled with clarity and insight.

Now relax and remove your focus from the serpent. You know it will take some time before the snake makes it to the next chakra, so you let it proceed at its own pace as you relax. Do not attempt to return the Kundalini serpent into a sleeping state; now that it is awake, you must not attempt to repress its growth.

Take three deep breaths, and open your eyes when you are ready.

During the next week or month, focus on your psychic self and how you use your abilities to understand the subtleties of the world around you. Do you listen to yourself or do you shrug off your psychic intuition as "Oh, it's nothing"? Give more credence to your ability to ferret out the truth of matters.

Awakening the Kundalini: Step Seven

Focus on your seventh chakra, resting on the top of your head. This is your crown chakra, which integrates every part of your being. It is here that you center yourself and find yourself in balance and harmony with the universe. Examine your seventh chakra carefully. Is it glowing a clear, pure light and swirling clockwise? If not, you will want to clear it.

Imagine a bright and sparkling diamond in your hand. Place the diamond against the chakra and feel it slip into the vortex in your body. Once inside, the diamond begins to burrow through your chakra, clearing out old gunk and debris. See memories of times you felt fragmented, times you felt out of balance with the universe and all that is part of it. See memories of points in your life when you didn't know who you were or why you were here. See all these thoughts and memories turn to dust and sweep out of your chakra on a sparkling crystal wind.

Imagine your chakra beginning to whirl in a clockwise motion, slowly at first, then faster and faster as the diamond cleans it out. The color flickers and turns into a clear, bright light, and you can feel yourself letting go of old feelings of alienation, of insecurity and fragmentation.

Now, see a coiled serpent resting in your sixth chakra; your Kundalini is waiting for your signal. The energy from the diamond shoots in a brilliant line and falls upon the serpent's face. One eye slowly opens, and then the other. The snake raises its head, and you can sense that it needs to stretch.

Watch as it raises up, slowly stretching its sinuous body as it flickers its tongue in and out of its mouth. It tastes the energy of your seventh chakra and very slowly begins to climb toward the vortex, searching, awakening sensations you never knew you had.

When it reaches your crown, you find yourself overwhelmed by the macrocosm of the universe, and within the macrocosm, that you sense the microcosm too—as above, so below. Inner/outer, infinite/finite, deity/mortal, fire/water, yin/yang, male/female. Everything is connected, even in their opposition, and you are a part of everything.

Take a moment to examine how it feels to be in balance with the universe, to be connected, a vital spark in the fires of life, and yet separate and unique.

Now relax and remove your focus from the serpent. The Kundalini has fully awakened and activated your chakras. You must never attempt to return the Kundalini serpent into a sleeping state; now that it is awake, you must not attempt to repress your growth and exploration.

Take three deep breaths, and open your eyes when you are ready.

During the next week or month, focus on your connection with all that exists. Listen to your heart, to your body, to your intuition and walk in balance, for you are a part of this universe, this world, this life. You are both a cosmic dust speck and a vital spark in the vastness of the universe.

Masturbation and Magic

Magical practitioners can use the energy of orgasm in several ways. I've found the following to be the most magical methods when working alone.

First, you need to have a focus for your magic. Casting a spell for yourself is a much better choice than casting for someone else. If you use your orgasmic energy to empower a spell for someone else, you run the risk of keying your sexual energy into their lives and this can have some interesting ramifications—from a mild flirtation springing up to outright obsession. Good subjects for spellcasting while using masturbation magic are self-esteem spells, beauty spells, personal power spells, love spells (not focused on any particular person), movement and exercise spells, and so on. In other words, personal body and emotional spells are your best choices.

I usually use candle magic when I'm working with sex magic; the candle's flame seems to mirror the heat of the passion. Other forms of magic will also work. Don't be shy, experiment.

Choose a candle, preferably an image candle (a yoni or lingam candle to match your gender), but a taper candle or votive will also provide a good effect. You may wish to perform the first steps in preparation a day before casting the spell. Anoint the candle thoroughly with your vaginal juices or semen. Give the candle a good coating and let it dry. This is the best binding you can use on a candle for sex magic spellwork.

On the day you wish to cast your spell, carve the candle with runes appropriate for the type of magic you are working with. For beauty runes, you might wish to use the Hathor rune (she is the Egyptian goddess of beauty and competent career women) or the rune of her mirror for beauty. For love, you have several rune choices: for sex and passion, the Norse bind rune is a good one to use.

A note about love magic: Never cast a spell onto one person in particular; you're asking for trouble if you do. Always cast a spell asking the universe or the gods to bring you whoever is right for you. This negates the chance for backlash in your spellwork and opens the way for the person who will be your proper match to enter your life. Trust me on this one; I've done it the other way and been burned. When I cast a love spell asking for the "right person," I met Samwise. I've never been disappointed with our match, even though it meant that I had to give up reeling in anyone else I attracted. (Lust magic and its results can be addictive. I've altered the focus to glamour magic to bring out the best in me, rather than to attract new men and women into my love life.)

After you've carved both your runes and the words for whatever you want to invoke on your candle, anoint it with either a few drops of your blood or magical oils. The magical oils should be geared toward the energy of the spell. Love, Lust, Come and See Me, personal power oils—any of these will work depending on what your focus is. After your candle is oiled, you can add extra energy if you like by rolling it in a magical powder. Remember, it's less expensive and much more effective to make the oils and powders yourself. A number of books, including my other books, provide instructions for making oil blends and powders.

Set your candle in a firm stable holder. Place it in a safe place in your bedroom (or wherever you're planning on casting your spell). If you want to set up an altar, use scarves and things that will mirror what you are trying to accomplish—color coordinate to the appropriate energy.

Building an altar can be a very creative way to infuse power into a ritual. As you add each object to your altar, focus on what it means to you and why you want to include it. For beauty, love, and lust magic, you might want to drape the table or shelf in pearls, gemstone necklaces, scarves, and perfume bottles. I raise energy and charge all my beauty supplies on a regular basis. Vanity? Perhaps, but the better we feel about ourselves, the more confident we are in all parts of our lives. For a more in-depth study of this issue, see my sister book, *Crafting the Body Divine*.

I find it best, for sex magic, to actually go ahead and cast a Circle and invoke the elements. This not only concentrates the energy, it keeps any nasty astral buggers out when you are in a vulnerable state of mind.

Invoke whichever god or goddess you have decided to work with, if you want to work with any. Be sure and do your research thoroughly, especially when working with sex magic. If you are a man with very few bisexual or gay tendencies, Pan might not be your best choice; you might want to invoke Cernunnos or Frey instead. If you are a woman and you invoke Pombagira, remember that she is the patron of prostitutes, transsexuals, and homosexuals. Is this the energy you had in mind? If so, great! If not, think twice.

I play music to fit the mood of the energy that I'm focusing on. I also find that dancing builds up a lot of sensuous energy and contributes to the overall rise in my power and passion.

Turn on your music, light your candle, and spend a little time sliding into the mindset for what you are doing. If it helps, read erotica, watch an X-rated movie, whatever it takes to get you going. Use fantasy but be careful; don't get caught up in sending the energy to the fantasy instead of to the spell.

I find the best way to counter this possibility is to fantasize with a focus on your spellwork. If it's for love, imagine being with someone whom you can love and be loved by (once again, try to make the individual a composite, not an actual person). If your spell is meant to enhance your passion and erotic nature, then fantasize about what you'd like to have happen in your sex life and the energy you'd like to radiate. If you are casting a spell for beauty and personal power, see yourself as you'd like to be (be realistic here, people; enhancement is the key, not plastic surgery).

When you begin to masturbate, try to focus on your spell. Use the plateau method we discussed earlier to build up energy. When you are at the point where you can't stop yourself—when you are going to climax—then send the energy rushing toward your magical objective.

Rest in the energy a while before you get up and devoke the elements and deities. Let your candle burn all the way out (it's easiest to put it in the bathroom away from any flammables, in a heatproof container in the tub) and then dispose of the wax remnants.

You can also use this magical technique to charge an herbal charm, though I would recommend wearing it in a sachet around your neck while you are raising energy and masturbating.

The magical energy we use in spellcasting is directly connected to the energy of the Kundalini. The two are entwined in a way we can not fully understand, but we can make use of that connection in our magic and in our passionate selves.

Masturbation is not only normal, it's healthy. Regular orgasms help keep our skin clear, our minds at peace, our bodies happy. When we mix masturbation with magic, we have an incredible recipe for personal power and strength. Don't let anyone tell you that pleasuring yourself is wrong. Be proud of your ability to give yourself such a wonderful gift. After all, if you can't enjoy your body, how can you expect anybody else to pleasure you? Love yourself, and you will be able to love more fully, on both a physical and an emotional basis.

CHAPTER FOUR

Fantasy and the Toy Box

Phebe: Good shepherd, tell this youth what 'tis to love
Silvius: It is to be all made of sighs and tears . . .
It is to be all made of faith and service . . .
It is to be all made of fantasy,
All made of passion, and all made of wishes

WILLIAM SHAKESPEARE, *As You Like It*

When you were a child, chances are you had a toy box. Now that you're grown, the toy box takes on a different meaning altogether. And the toys—well, we aren't playing with Barbie and GI Joe dolls anymore. We're still buying batteries, but not for a remote-controlled car.

Sex toys can elicit a lot of laughter and embarrassment. They're still associated with dark seedy stores where nasty men in raincoats hang out. However, with chain stores like Lovers Package and women-run shops like Toys in Babeland, the sex shop has come into its own. Airy and bright, many of these new stores are organized like any specialty boutique, and the clerks are usually friendly and knowledgeable about their products. Some stores offer workshops on various aspects of sexuality, and some shops are oriented toward women and couples.

So what is a sex toy? Simply put, it is an object used during sex for sexual pleasure. The list is as varied as the people who buy them. Sexual toys could even include an address book and a steno book if you want to play "boss and secretary" role-playing games.

The most common sex toys found in sex shops are vibrators and dildos. These are mainly used for vaginal and anal insertion and clitoral stimulation, though some men enjoy the feeling of a vibrator pressed against their penis or scrotum. What's the difference between a dildo and a vibrator? Dildos usually don't have a motor and are used on a manual basis, while vibrators have a battery- or electric-operated motor, which makes them vibrate at varying speeds, from slow to extremely fast.

Dildos have been around since prehistoric times. Phallic-shaped batons have been discovered in Upper Paleolithic art. The English word *dildo* dates back to at least the 1500s. In ancient Greece, they were called *olisbos* and were made from wood or soft leather. They were quite popular in Egypt, China, and other parts of Asia. Today, some of the most popular dildos are silicone based, and they feel remarkably fleshlike. Crystal batons are becoming popular, though I wonder whether they aren't more of an art statement rather than serving any functional purpose. There are the ever-popular metal dildos too; however, metal is more popular for vibrators.

Vibrators come in two types: electric and battery operated. The electric ones tend to be quieter, have more intensity, and of course, they don't run out of juice. However, you have to be near an outlet, and the vibrations can be too intense for some women. Battery-operated vibrators are portable and louder, but work pretty well. I recommend a battery charger in order to be kind to the environment. Once you get into using a vibrator, you'll find you become the battery salesman's best friend.

Vibrators and dildos come in all shapes and sizes, from tiny egg-shaped ones for clitoral stimulation (these are wonderful, folks), to huge cock-shaped dildos with a texture like real skin. You like hot pink? There are hot pink vibrators. You want something shaped like a cucumber? There's a cucumber-shaped one. There are also remote-controlled vibrators for those of you who want to give someone else the chance to play with you.

If the sensations are too intense against your clitoris, then try a thin towel or piece of cloth between you and the vibrator. Test several varieties. You can never have too many toys. Their durability depends on the amount of use they get and whether you drop them on the floor or a hard surface. Battery-operated vibrators typically wear out after a short time so don't feel embarrassed or that you're masturbating with them too much; it's the manufacturer's fault, not yours.

Clitoral vibrators are a lot of fun. Often shaped like an egg or sometimes like a small animal (yeah, that does seem odd, but you will get over the "this is weird" feeling pretty fast), these little gems are incredibly effective. Their use is enhanced by using a dildo in your vagina while pressing the vibrator against your clit. Or you can use the vibrator during sex if your partner doesn't object.

Ben wa balls will have the same effect as a dildo during your fun time. The subject of some controversy, they are usually either loved or discarded totally. Two metal balls about the size of Ping-Pong balls, they are often attached to one another on a string. You insert them in the vagina and, as you walk, dance, or what have you, they move gently, producing some interesting sensations. They can be fun to include in B&D scenes. Again, it's a matter of what works for you.

Cock rings encircle the cock, and sometimes the balls, and they promote longer erections by restricting blood flow out of the erection. The main concern here is that you shouldn't leave it on for more than twenty minutes at a time. There have been cases where men ended up in the hospital, unable to remove the ring (usually the ones without snaps). As with any device that slows down the supply of blood flow, use your common sense. However, with proper use, men tend to report that cock rings really enhance their enjoyment and arousal.

Artificial vaginas are fleshlike sheaths that fit tightly over an erect penis and are used for male masturbation. They can be ribbed or lubricated and come in varying sizes for your personal tastes. Artificial dolls also serve this purpose, simulating oral, anal, and vaginal sex for men.

Anal plugs are usually tapered with a flared base. They are inserted into the anus, and they stimulate the sensitive nerve endings in the rectum. Available in varying sizes and shapes, they are often used in kink. Some have a tail attached to them so they look like a pony's tail. These are typically used in training pony girls and boys.

Nipple clamps generally fall under two categories: alligator clips (which have a screw to adjust the pressure) and tweezer clips, which act like tweezers to pinch the nipple. Most nipple clips have a chain connecting the two clips. These are generally used for kink, too, though variations are popular now in nipple piercing.

Blindfolds, wrist cuffs, and leg cuffs are used during bondage play. I prefer leather and suede wrist cuffs that have buckles. Velcro seems a bit silly to me, though some people will be more comfortable with its easy release. I like my wrist cuffs strong and secure, with hoops that allow chains or ropes to connect the pair.

Silk and velvet scarves can be used for bondage too. Samwise and I have a crushed velvet belt that we use in our practice, and we use pretty swag lamp hooks screwed into the wall at the head of the bed to hook the wrist cuffs or scarf on when my hands are tied. By the way, serious bondage aficionados seldom use real handcuffs. They cut into the wrists. Leather or other soft wrist and ankle cuffs are a much better choice.

In advanced bondage play, a gag, harness, or leash may also be used, but these are better left until you have more experience.

Flails can be as soft as a gentle whisper or as harsh as a leather strap, depending on what you prefer. If you choose to delve into sadomasochism, please read some good texts on the subject and discuss it with others in the BDSM community to learn how to effectively use a whip, flail, or cane. I have listed some very good references in the bibliography for your interest.

Feathers can be used to tickle and tease. Ostrich and peacock feathers are your best choices. Oils are nice, not only for lubrication, but also for erotic massage and grooming. Kama Sutra makes a lovely line of edible oils and balms that enhance pleasure when you apply them to nipples and genitals by (depending on the product) gently numbing the area with a cool mint feeling and taste or warming it up with a cinnamon flavor. If you use magical oils in your sex magic practices, make sure they don't include more than a few drops of hot oils, such as cinnamon, which can burn the body, and for gods' sake, *don't* eat them! Most magical oils contain ingredients that are somewhat poisonous if not downright deadly. On the other hand, body paints are usually edible or can be used in the bathtub as soap. Read the package for instructions. These can be a fun addition to your toy box.

Food has long been used during sex. Whipped cream, flavored syrups, fruits, you name it, someone has probably found an erotic use for it. Ideally, you will keep your food in your refrigerator, not in your toy box. Don't be afraid to experiment, just make sure that if you use some sort of food as a dildo, you clean yourself thoroughly afterward to avoid infection.

Always clean any toy that touches your genitals every time you use it— you don't want bacteria to grow and give you an oh-so-not-fun infection. Baby wipes work well for this and are easy to keep by the bed. Also, and this is very important in both masturbation and sexual intercourse, anything, be it vibrator or penis, that enters your anus, should be cleaned *before* it is inserted into your vagina. Your vaginal bacteria won't upset your anal passage, but your anal bacteria can cause an infection in your vagina. If you're having anal sex, insist on a new condom after anal intercourse even if your partner hasn't come yet. You should keep yourself in good condition, both internally and externally.

You might want to buy a pretty box for your toys—doesn't your sex life deserve to be treated with respect and admiration, rather than hiding its paraphernalia in the closet or under your undies in your dresser drawer? Of course, if you are underage and you don't want your folks to find out you own a vibrator, then you might want to keep it safely out of sight.

Fantasy's Role in Sexuality

The brain is the biggest sex organ, and fantasy is an integral part of human nature. Until the last decade or so in our modern society, it was assumed that women did not fantasize. Men bought porn and this was accepted, at least for bachelors. However, no one really paid attention to all those romance novels that millions of women bought and read. The truth was ignored in the effort to maintain the pretense that "nice girls don't have sex, fantasize, masturbate, hold hard-edged careers, fill in the blank."

As a writer, I can guarantee you that these bodice rippers and historical romances may occasionally have good plots, but women weren't and aren't devouring them by the hundreds for plot alone. We are talking soft-core pornography here, erotica for women who had and have no other way to express their sexual desires. When reading romance novels, women can imagine themselves in the heroine's place and go on wild journeys of fantasy. All the elements are there: the dashing hero and the damsel in distress, the harem and the sultan, the pirates and the lady stolen away from her husband, the governess and the master.

When Nancy Friday made history with the publication of her book, *My Secret Garden: Women's Sexual Fantasies*, a compendium of women's fantasies that she had collected, it shook up established views on women and their tendency to fantasize, including those who insisted that women do not fantasize. All of a sudden, men were looking at their wives, their sisters, their friends, and mothers with new eyes. These women were kinky! We learned that women were fantasizing not only about sleeping with their husband's best friend, but with his wife, too. Women were contemplating their German shepherds with open lust; they were eyeing their son's friends with desire. Women, it seemed, were longing for the passion that they didn't receive at home.

When I read *My Secret Garden* and *Forbidden Flowers*, one thing I noted over and over again was the number of letters that started out with a resigned acceptance of being in a bad sexual relationship. The husband either didn't enjoy sex, didn't want to try anything new, or didn't care about the woman's sexual pleasure.

It's partly true that modern women have allowed this to happen, but prior to the 1980s and 1990s, women have had little choice in the matter. With the lack of good jobs for women, they were often totally dependent on their husbands' salaries. How could one support four children on welfare? And the social stigma of divorce was intense. When women complained to their doctors about their dissatisfaction with their lives, they were often given prescriptions for Valium to calm them down. The Rolling Stones didn't write *Mother's Little Helper* without inspiration. Prescriptions for Valium were handed out like candy to make sure women quietly, docilely accepted their place.

Don't get me wrong here. Antidepressants and sedatives can be useful and medically warranted. However, medicating to repress natural tendencies or to avoid coping with real concerns can have serious repercussions.

During the past two decades there has, indeed, been a shift. Women are demanding more. We want better jobs, better pay, more respect and more sexual satisfaction. Ms. Friday substantiates this in her book *Women on Top: How Real Life Has Changed Women's Fantasies*. These fantasies are more assertive and graphic than in her earlier books.

We do not have to settle for bad sex, no sex, or boring sex. However, what we want in fantasy is not always something we want in reality. In a fantasy you are in complete control of everyone's actions. You alone control the scene. In reality, we do not and cannot control our partners. Real life is not like a play or a film. Even if partners agree to stick to a script, we can't always guarantee that they'll do so with the same energy with which we invest them in our fantasies. Sometimes things are better left to our imagination. I may have fantasies of sleeping with two or more men at the same time, but I'm not going to act on them because I cannot control the actions of my partners and I'm married and in a monogamous relationship. If I were single, my decision might be different.

Tips for Fantasizing without Guilt

Fantasy can include anything from a passing thought about the woman who walks by your desk to an intricate and complex play-by-play movie while you're masturbating. Your sexual fantasies can increase your pleasure, and therefore make you happier with your sex life, which will enhance your relationship.

However, you must accept that your partner is most likely fantasizing, too. You may want to sit down and discuss the role of fantasy in your relationship, but it may not be a good idea to share your wilder fantasies unless you are very secure with your partnership. I used to feel threatened that Samwise might be fantasizing about other women until I forced myself to accept that I was fantasizing about both other men and other women. I would have been guilty of a double standard had I not acknowledged that what was normal for me was also normal for him and that our fantasies would not interfere with our love and desire for each other.

You may want to read or view some erotica or pornography to stimulate your imagination if you have trouble allowing yourself to create your own fantasies. There is a lot of controversy over pornography and whether or not it degrades women. I have to state that, as a writer, I can not condone censorship. While I find some pornography disturbing, I do enjoy erotica, so I'm not going to judge anything out there that meets the legal requirements (in other words, *no* kiddy porn, snuff films, or forced participation).

As to whether porn sparks unacceptable behavior and standards, well, I think that a lot of the actual perverts out there would behave the same way if they didn't have access to porn. Porn may suggest impossible standards for women, but fashion magazines do the same thing and, in many cases, are worse culprits than a girlie mag.

Think of fantasy as an exercise for your imagination. You might want to write down some of your favorites in a private journal. You may find that you replay certain scenarios over and over again, while others pass on without incident.

If you have a repeating fantasy that you would like to experience, broach partner about acting it out. Don't press the issue if your partner is uncomfortable with it. You can, however, discuss what makes them hesitant and possibly create an acceptable compromise. When you bring fantasy to reality, remember that it will never be quite the same in practice as it is in thought. It might be better or not as good. Manifesting a fantasy is bound to be fraught with alterations.

A simple and silly example is that when Samwise started tying me up, I didn't count on the fact that when my nose itched it was ridiculously distracting. All of a sudden, I had to ask him to scratch my nose since my hands were hooked up to the wall. In a sense, it reinforced the restraint aspect and made it more exciting.

Another time, his blood sugar started to drop, and I had to make sure he untied me so I could get him enough food to prevent him from slipping into a diabetic seizure. Now we always make sure that I can get the knots in the scarf undone or the cuffs off should an emergency arise. We also make sure that he eats before we have any intensive sex play. It's a necessary compromise for our particular situation.

Some Common and Not-So-Common Fantasies

Think your fantasies are wild and out of control? Not likely. Just about anything is fair game for fantasy, and there's nothing wrong with letting your imagination go wild. Whips, chains, wrist cuffs, scarves, feathers, hot wax.

If you can imagine it, you can fantasize about it. To give you an idea, here are some of the more common themes found in fantasies:

- Having sex with someone other than your partner. Most often the stranger will be a "forbidden" person—your husband's best friend, your wife's hairstylist.

- Multiple partners. This fantasy is common among both men and women. The most common fantasy for men is having sex with two women at one time; for women, two or more men at the same time raises its kinky head. Orgies straight out of *Caligula* are not out of the ordinary in our X-rated theater of the mind.

- Role-playing fantasies. These include the slave girl and the sultan, the dominatrix and the slave boy, the school girl and the headmaster, the French maid and the master, strangers meeting in a bar, and so on.

- "Sweep me away" fantasies. These are often used to alleviate guilt. These are fantasies in which the sexual encounter is forced, so it's not your fault. These fantasies should never be confused with fantasies of actual rape. The scene is completely controlled by the person fantasizing and is in no way like the reality of being forced into sex. I speak from experience.

- Fantasies involving homosexual encounters. Both men and women admit to gay or lesbian fantasies, whether or not they have a natural bent for that gender preference. However, on the whole, women seem less reluctant to discuss these fantasies and more interested in trying them out in real life. A surprising number of men get turned on by imagining two women fucking each other. I know that when I was with my girlfriend, we had a lot of guys on our tails, trying to get an invitation to our bedroom.

⇨ Bestiality fantasies. There are a number of women who fantasize about having sex with dogs, horses, and snakes. The connection between women and their love for horses has long been seen as a metaphor for their desire for sex. Men seem to fantasize about watching women having sex with animals. When played out in reality, this definitely falls under the section of kink. I personally don't think any animal should be forced into a sexual situation with a human being, but I won't say it's "wrong" when used as a fantasy tool.

Whether or not we find any of these desires disgusting or exciting, we must accept that, in fantasy, anything goes and one person's pleasure may be another person's nightmare. Choose your dreams carefully; sometimes we actually get what we think we want.

CHAPTER FIVE

Sheelah Na Gigs and Sacred Harlots

My vulva, the horn,
The Boat of Heaven,
Is full of eagerness like the young moon.
As for me, Inanna,
Who will plow my vulva?
Who will plow my high field?
Who will plow my wet ground?

Great Lady, the king will plow your vulva.
I, Dumuzi the King, will plow your vulva.

SUMERIAN HYMN FOR INANNA

The Great Rite. The Hieros Gamos. Called by many names, it is the connection of the divine to the divine, of god to goddess, of the ruler of the land to the Earth. It is the union of opposites, polarities blending even as they conflict, yin and yang. It is the sacred marriage. The rut of the King Stag embodies the strength of the God; the open, yielding darkness into which he thrusts is the dark cavern of the Great Mother. Together they unite to create life.

Sheelah Na Gig

The Sheelah Na Gigs are figures found throughout western Europe and the United Kingdom. A bas relief set in stone, the Sheelah usually portrays a naked woman holding her genitals spread wide and is thought possibly (though the origin is uncertain) to date back to the time of Sumer, where the women of the temple were known as *nu-gigs*, meaning "pure" or "spotless." According to Barbara Walker, the word *gig* also means female genitals and might be connected to the Irish *jig*, which in turn is linked to the French word *gigue*, meaning an orgiastic pre-Christian dance.

Some Sheelahs have skull-like heads, others are grimacing and leering. All are considered rather crude or lewd. We find them on cathedrals and churches, along with Green Man statues (statues of male fertility). They are the God and Goddess making themselves known even through the customs of the new religion and Christian veneer painted over the old holidays.

It is likely that they relate directly to the Celtic goddesses, most of whom had a dual nature. Sexuality and fierceness were linked. Throughout the centuries, the figures have come to be talismans and charms.

The Sacred Harlots of the Goddess

Before sex was considered a sin, the Sacred Harlot held a place of prominence and importance in many cultures. The etymology of the words *whore* and *harlot* show this lineage. The *horeae* were multicultural in origin. Known as *houris* in Persia, they were *harines* in Babylon, and ladies of the hour in Egypt. In Greece, they became Aphrodite's celestial nymphs. Harlot priestesses, these women also acted as midwives and healers and trained men in sexual mysteries. *Horology*, which means timekeeping, is based on the systems designed by these priestesses.

We also find that the *hora*, a Jewish dance, is based on the dances of the sacred harlots.

Merlin Stone (author of *When God Was a Woman*) notes that the Hebrew word *zonah* refers to both prostitute and prophetess. *Puta*, the Spanish word for whore, has its beginnings in the Latin *puticuli*, which derives from hole in the earth, the womb of rebirth. In turn, *puticuli* is rooted in the Vedic *puta*, meaning "pure" or "holy."

When Christianity took over, Ishtar, the Great Mother of the Babylonians, became known as the Great Whore of Babylon. The fathers of the church declared her sexuality and her very existence to be sinful, but her worship and influence were not easily destroyed. Also known as Har, the Lady of Harlots, she was beloved by those who lived in her lands. Ishtar was a multifaceted goddess who touched every part of daily life. Her priestesses were considered prophets and healers, as well as sexual ritualists.

The Code of Hammurabi, which limited women's rights in some spheres, protected the sacred whores or harlots from slander and upheld the rights of their children. They could inherit property and receive income; essentially their reputations were as worthy as those of a married woman. Though special housing was set aside for Ishtar's whores, they were free to live where they wished. However, they could not open "wine shops" if they lived outside the designated housing, nor could they enter a tavern, presumably to separate them from "common" prostitutes.

During this time, every woman in Babylon was required to serve a term in the temples of Ishtar, when she would have sexual intercourse with any stranger who requested her. No woman refused, for it was a transgression against the Goddess to ignore her edict. A man would walk through the temple and make his choice. He would toss the required coins in the woman's lap and say, "May the Goddess Mylitta make thee happy." The woman would offer the coins to the Goddess and lie with the man, after which she was released from her duty. She would return to the temple daily until she had serviced one man.

By the third century B.C.E., as we saw in chapter 1, when the Akkadians conquered Sumer, sacred prostitution became a shameful profession. The most likely theory is that, along with the rise of a system as patriarchal as this one was, knowledge of paternity became much more important, and women's sexual freedom was restricted. Joseph Campbell, however, in *The Masks of God: Occidental Mythology*, proposes that: "the power of this goddess-mother of the world overthrown by her sons" reflected a mass Oedipal complex that turned men against the freer spirits of women.

Cunti, an Oriental goddess known as the yoni of the universe, is the source of a number of our words today, including the infamous word *cunt*. The meaning was synonymous with "woman" and was not meant to be derogative. *Cunning* and *kenning* also come from her name, as do *cunicle* (a passageway) and *cunabula* (a cradle). We find her reflected in Cunina, a Roman goddess who protected children, and in Kundah, a Saharan goddess of the Kuntah tribe who ascribed their origins to "the cleft of the Goddess." Cunti or Kunda was also the title used for Kali-Ma, Black Mother of India, who is a consort to Shiva and is connected to Shakti, the Hindu goddess of sexuality.

The Sacred Harlot's Purpose

The purpose of the sacred whore, or harlot, was far more than to be a woman who sexually serviced men. She acted as go-between, a representative of the Goddess in mortal form so men might commune and join with the divine through sexual activity. She was also a conduit for prophecy and healing. The women who served as priestesses of these goddesses were respected for their office. They were seen as sacred emissaries and were highly trained in their arts. Men came to them in reverence, not anger, in a desire for a divine connection, not just to get laid. Do not confuse a woman who served in Ishtar's service with a common streetwalker. They were on very different levels and were treated with consideration and respect, not with contempt.

When the Great Rite is performed by Pagans today, it's a reenactment of this communion. The priest approaches the priestess with reverence, for she is the altar of the goddess, she is the goddess incarnate.

And though I firmly believe that you can practice sex magic and reach the divine through both homosexual experience and masturbation, I think the strongest connection is made through the pairing of male and female. This union joins opposites, and it provides the connection that can spark conception and life. I believe that possibility, that conjunction of energies, most fully explores the divine marriage, the Great Rite.

I also believe the ritual can work in reverse. When the woman assumes the role of the Sacred Harlot and the man approaches her seeking the divine, she guides him to communion with the goddess. Similarly, the man can play the Stag King, and guide a woman to a sacred connection with the Horned God. There are many cases in aboriginal cultures that show a woman being married to an icon of a god, often in the form of a large phallic standing stone, pole, or tree.

Having said that, it's interesting to note how many Pagans I've met (including myself) who are bisexual. There is also a fairly large gay population within the Pagan community. I believe that Paganism allows us the freedom to fully explore our sexuality without the feelings of guilt that traditional mores and values tend to instill.

Becoming the Sacred Harlot: An Autoerotic Ritual for Women

For your ritual, select the day of a full or new moon, depending on whether you want to invoke the Goddess as Bright Mother or as the Dark Lady. Be sure that you are comfortable touching your body. If you do not feel comfortable with this, then study chapter 3 and practice those exercises until you can give yourself an orgasm with ease and without guilt.

Spend several days preparing for this ritual. You should do this in a leisurely fashion; rush nothing during this time. Gather the following items:

- bath salts—rose or vanilla works best. Or use perfumed bath gel instead. If not allergic, add incense or potpourri to match.

- a candle. If you can obtain a red female-image candle or a yoni-shaped candle, do so. Otherwise, use a red votive or taper candle. Anoint it with a magical oil like Come to Me, or a lust oil. You might also wish to use my Intoxication Oil (the recipe follows at the end of this chapter). Anoint the candle with your vaginal juices.

- lingerie, something that makes you feel sensual and passionate. No flannel here; wear lace or satin, whatever sparks off your fingertips when you touch your skin beneath the negligee.

- several magazines with images that reflect your idea of sexuality: the sacred, passionate, dark depths of your being. The day before your ritual, cut sexy, sensual images from these magazines and glue them on a poster board creating a collage. Hang it in a private space where it can spark your sense of yourself as sexy and vibrant. For more information on creative collage, see my book *Embracing the Moon*.

- your favorite sex toys.

The day before your ritual, clean your bedroom and arrange to have several hours free from interruption. Tape record the meditation. It's much more effective if you have it on cassette.

On the day of the ritual, prepare a light snack of your choice of the following: fruit, chocolate, cookies, cheese, and wine or grape juice. You might choose chocolate-dipped strawberries, Colby, and a sweet Riesling. Light the incense in your room and place your collage where you can see it. Take a leisurely ritual bath with the bath salts or gel. When you are finished, gently towel off and slip into your lingerie. Return to your room. Then cast a Circle and call on the elements in a manner similar to this:

I cast this Circle once round in the name of the Maiden, who takes joy in her own body, who is the face of the Goddess unleashed, who is she who owns herself and no man may enter her garden, but only her own hand.

I cast this Circle twice round in the name of the Mother, who is in full blossom in her sexuality, who is the face of the Goddess unmatched, who is she who gives and receives from others. Only those may enter her garden who can give pleasure as well as take from the bloom.

I cast this Circle thrice round in the name of the Crone, who is the culmination of experience, who is the face of the Goddess untamed. I call to she who teaches the arts of love to those who are new to the embrace of passion. Only those may enter her garden who are willing to learn.

Next invoke the elements. Turn to the north, and say:

Spirits of the Earth, I call thee forth to attend my ritual. Rise up thickly through my feet, you who are the roots of this world, you who are bone and stone and crystal and branch. Ground me into the energy of my body, that I might commune with the Divine through touch and sense and feeling. Spirits of the Earth, manifest in me the Sacred Harlot of the Goddess, that I might wear the cloak of her being, so that I might express the earthiness of her essence. Welcome, Spirits of the Earth, and Blessed Be.

Turn to the east, and say:

Spirits of the Wind, I call thee forth to attend my ritual. Sweep through my body, you who are mist and vapor, you who are cloud and wind and fog and storm. Remove stagnation and bring a clarity to my spirit, that I might commune with the Divine through spirit and soul and illumination. Spirits of the Wind, manifest in me the Sacred Harlot of the Goddess, that I might wear the cloak of her being, so that I might express the brilliance of her mind. Welcome, Spirits of the Wind, and Blessed Be.

Turn to the south, and say:

Spirits of the Flame, I call thee forth to attend my ritual. Burn through my loins, you who are flame and fire, you who are the golden sun, the glowing lava, the rising Phoenix. Pull me into the trance, into the dance, that I might commune with the Divine through my passion. Spirits of the Flame, manifest in me the Sacred Harlot of the Goddess, that I might wear the cloak of her being, so that I might express the passion of her sexuality. Welcome, Spirits of the Flame, and Blessed Be.

Turn to the west, and say:

Spirits of the Water, I call thee forth to attend my ritual. Flow through my heart and soul, you who are the raging river, the crashing ocean breakers, the still pool of the grotto. Lead me into the core of my being, into the hidden depths of my soul, that I might commune with the Divine through my love and my sorrow. Spirits of the Water, manifest in me the Sacred Harlot of the Goddess, that I might wear the cloak of her being, so that I might express the joy in her heart. Welcome, Spirits of the Water, and Blessed Be.

Light your candle and invoke one of the goddesses who was worshiped by the sacred whores. I suggest Ishtar; she is far safer to invoke than Kali-Ma. Or you may wish to call upon Aphrodite or Inanna. Do a bit of research and adjust the following invocation appropriately:

Mighty Ishtar, the Great Har of Babylon, I call to thee. Oh, Great Mother, come to me for this ritual. Invest in me the feeling of your

102

*sacred sexuality; let me understand my connection to you, to my essence
as Woman, through this ritual and rite. Be with me as I explore the
realms of my sex, as I explore what it means to be part of the Goddess,
the eternal and divine nature of the feminine. Ishtar, Mother of
Civilization, come to me and be with me. Welcome, Gracious Lady,
and Blessed Be.*

When you have invoked the Goddess, turn on your favorite sensual
music and begin to explore your body. The meditation will come a bit later.
First, make yourself comfortable as you lull yourself into a sensual trance.
Drink a bit of the wine or grape juice, and feel it slide down your throat.
How does it feel? Is it smooth? Is it fiery?

Now lay on your bed or stand in front of your mirror and begin to caress
your body. Run your hands lightly over your breasts and watch your
nipples stand erect. Pinch them, play with them. Let your mind revel in the
sensations you are feeling.

Sway to the music. Visualize a temple dance; you are dancing for the
Goddess. Let yourself go. There is no one to watch or judge you. As you
dance, caress yourself, run your hands over your arms, up and down your
legs, through your hair. Lose yourself in the music, lose yourself in the
magic of your passion and desire.

When you are aroused, take three deep breaths and let yourself plateau.
Settle into this new level of awareness, and turn off the music. Slip your cassette of the meditation in, and lay down on your bed. Follow the words of
the meditation as you use your vibrator or hand to pleasure yourself and
bring yourself to orgasm. Focus on the meditation, and channel the passion
that builds into those thoughts.

Meditation for a Sacred Harlot Ritual

Take three deep breaths. You are standing in a large open room that
is filled with silken pillows and long velveteen drapes trimmed with

gold cording. You are clad in a long brocade dress, and you know you are in the Temple of Ishtar to serve as a sacred harlot. *(pause)*

Three women come in and lead you to an inner chamber. You see a square pool in the center of the chamber, filled with steaming water and rose petals. The women remove your clothes and set them carefully to one side. They admire your body: one comments on the beauty of your skin, another runs her hand through your hair and tells you how pretty it is. Their touch feels good, and they encourage you to slip into the fragrant pool. *(pause)*

As you bathe, they wash your hair for you and pour steaming vats of perfumed water over your back. Luxuriate in the feeling as the liquid streams down your bare skin. *(extended pause—one minute)*

The women help you out of the pool and dry you with thick towels. One of them combs out your hair, carefully unknotting any tangles and gently drying your locks with another towel. *(pause)*

The second woman begins to rub your breasts and belly with an oil that smells of peaches and dark musk. Her hands glide over your flesh, cupping the curves, lingering in the hollows. The oil glistens on your skin like sweat. Can you sense the touch of her fingers on your skin? Run your hands down your body as you see her doing the same. *(pause)*

The third woman prepares a simple white linen dress for you to slip into. She slides it around your shoulders and ties it closed with a golden belt. The material feels soft against your skin, smooth, with no scratchy feel at all. *(pause)*

The women lead you out to a hallway that opens onto the temple's front steps. You can see olive trees in the distance, and date palms, and long, unending patches of sand. As you look around, you see other women sitting on the temple's steps, gently waving papyrus fans to stir a light breeze. One of the women points to an open spot and motions for you to sit and wait. *(pause)*

You have come to the temple this day, summoned by tradition. Every woman, married or unmarried, must spend one day of her life in service to Ishtar as a sacred harlot. This is your day. You feel a stir of pride inside your breast, even as your face flushes lightly. As you look around, you see men approaching women. Today, along with those other women, you stand as the Goddess. Today you will pleasure whichever man chooses you. You will approach him as a divine woman, sacred in your sexuality, and offer him the blessings of Ishtar through your body. *(extended pause—one minute)*

As the day passes, you begin to wonder whether you will have to return tomorrow, but as the sun creeps lower in the sky, you look up to see a man standing in front of you. He is of average height, with curly dark hair and a long beard. A sparkle in his eye borders on laughter as he drops a handful of coins in your lap. "May the goddess Mylitta make thee happy," he says and extends his hand. *(pause)*

You lead the man into the temple to the rooms set aside for sacred worship. Candlelight glistens against the silken draperies that cover the archway leading into the chamber, and a soft bed of embroidered brocade pillows lays across the floor. There is a bowl in which to place the offering of coins, and you drop them in as your gift to the

Goddess for serving her. Then you turn to the man and look into his eyes. *(pause)*

"I come seeking the Goddess," he says in a throaty voice. "I seek initiation into the secrets of her mysteries."

As you look at him, you see that more lies in his eyes than simple lust. You can feel his thirst to touch the Divine, to reach out, to make love to the Goddess, and it stirs a longing in you to fulfill that need and to lead him into the labyrinths of the Lady. *(pause)*

Slowly untie the cord that binds your dress to your waist and let the dress slip off your shoulders to the floor. As your garment falls away, the man watches you closely, and in his hungry stare, you feel beautiful. No matter what insecurities you may have had, no matter how tense you are about your body, this man makes you feel desirable. You hear him inhale sharply as the cool breeze wisps past your nipples, causing them to stiffen. *(pause)*

He takes a step forward and cautiously reaches out. "Oh, Lady, you are so beautiful, so lovely," he whispers. He pulls his hands back and then falls to his knees at your feet and lowers his head. "I do not deserve you," he says. "I am but a mortal man. I am fallible, coarse, and crude. How can you love me? How can you touch me without defiling your brilliance?" *(pause)*

As you stand there, gazing down at him, you feel a surge of love for this man, for all men. Yes, they can be coarse and crude, and all mortals have failings, but you also see into his heart. Ishtar shines through you like a glowing sun through a clear window, and you can read his soul. *(pause)*

When you look at him, you can see his childhood. His hands were slapped when he touched his penis; he was told he was dirty, he was wrong. You can feel the shame that he felt in his desire, and the pride he wanted to feel as his cock grew erect. You see him age a bit, and see him watching young women walk by. His loins burned, his heart raced—how much he wanted to reach out, to touch, to hold, to kiss. But again, he was turned away. Anger flared in his heart, but he realized that it wasn't the women he was angry at, but himself, for he still heard the words of his youth, "You've got a dirty mind; don't think that! Don't touch yourself!" (*pause*)

And now you see him, once again growing older. He found a small kitten, took it home to nurture it. You can sense the love he held for this animal, but his friends laughed at him for his gentleness. He kept the cat, but hid his feelings for it, sometimes even from himself. But late at night, when the tabby crawled on his chest, he petted it gently and crooned to it like he might to a child. (*pause*)

Now he seeks a mate, but you sense the ambiguity in his heart. He desires love and passion, yet he fears intimacy. He longs for closeness to the woman of his dreams, but fears she will be repulsed by his animal nature. He does not understand women, does not see that they, too, long for sex. That they, too, are insecure and ashamed of themselves. (*pause*)

You see all these things within him, and you feel a desire to heal this schism of feelings. Reach down; lift his chin up. There are tears in his eyes, and now, at your touch, they spill over onto his cheeks. "Come," you say, and take his hand to help him rise. You lead him over to the pile of pillows and face him, unashamed of your nakedness, for you feel truly embodied in the brilliance of Ishtar. Help him remove his clothes, piece by piece; reveal his body. *(pause)*

He is of average height, with a broad chest. Hair curls along his skin, and you can smell a whiff of musk as you trace his arms with your fingertips. As he drops his trousers, you look down to see his shaft thickening, rising under your watchful gaze. A tangle of curly hair surrounds his cock and balls, and a subtle thrill runs through you. Look again into his face. Even as his tears still flow, you see the grateful smile waiting for you, and a wave of desire sweeps over you. *(pause)*

"Touch me," you say. He lifts one hand to your waist, and pulls you close, into a tight embrace. His lips meet yours, and his tongue delves deeply into your mouth. A faint stirring of fire wells up in your belly, and you feel the Kundalini uncoil as the man's mouth presses more insistently on your own. You return his passion and slide your arms around him, drawing him down onto the bed. *(pause)*

He moans softly, slides his fingers along your leg, then reaches down to kiss your feet, your ankles, to work his way up along your inner thighs. You reach out again to touch him, but he pushes your hand gently away as he continues to trail kisses up your leg. "Let me worship you," he says. "Let me give unto you, my Lady." *(pause)*

With one hand, he pries your knees further apart, and you spread your legs. With his other hand, he slips into your sacred realm and runs his fingertips around the inside of your vagina. Moisture beads along his fingers, and as you shift under the pleasure that his slow, sensuous touch is giving you, he slides his fingers out and presses firmly on your clit. A ripple runs up your spine, up the Kundalini, into your breasts, and your breath becomes ragged. *(pause)*

He works you harder, then leans down and separates the folds of your labia. You can feel his hot breath as he extends his tongue, curls it around the your sacred lotus blossom, and begins to suck gently. A warm fluid starts to flow in your pussy as the tension mounts. The heat starts to build as he picks up the pace, licking, nipping. Let your body move, writhe against the insistence of his searching mouth. You are wet now, moister than you thought you could be, and a warm, musky scent rises up to you from this stranger who is now exploring you so intimately. *(pause)*

With a quick thrust, he slides his fingers inside you, driving them to a quick beat—faster, faster. A fire begins to build deep within your core, and it is like no fire you've felt before. This flame is fed from the flames of Ishtar; this fire is fed by the fuel of a Goddess. *(extended pause—one minute)*

You rise on his touch, wings taking hold of your breath and stealing it away. You feel as if you are soaring up a spiral staircase on golden clouds. Take three deep breaths, and let each breath lift you onto a new level of consciousness, a new height of awareness. *(pause)*

Now he shifts and slides up to face you. In his eyes, you see the light of a man who is experiencing something he has never felt—true acceptance of his masculinity and joy that a woman is taking such pleasure in his body. He whispers, "Thank you, thank you," as he burrows his nose into your neck, nibbling and licking your tender skin. He traces a line down your neck, over your shoulder, to your breast and takes one nipple in his mouth. *(pause)*

You can feel his energy, and you know how much he's enjoying himself, how much he likes hearing your moans of pleasure. As he enters you and begins to move, a sweep of light rushes through you, and Ishtar is fully within your heart, caring for this man, caring for you, enjoying the revelry of his body inside yours. You reach up, embrace him, and as you do so, you feel Ishtar embracing him, pulling her to him—man to woman, child to mother, student to teacher, devotee to goddess. She is all things, an overwhelming, consummate love, and she is within you and yet outside you at the same time. You can feel her love and radiance shine both for you and through you. *(extended pause—one minute)*

A light emanates from his eyes as he holds you in his embrace; his drive quickens, and you match the cadence. You sense a drumbeat in the distance, and you can feel the passion of every union that has ever been made with love and respect in the echo of your own cries. Quickly now, he thrusts within you, and quickly you return his fervor. *(pause)*

You see Ishtar standing beside you. As the man rears back, crying out, she reaches down and kisses his brow in a blessing. Then she turns to you and presses her lips against yours, and you feel how encompassing she is, how powerful and brilliant this ancient goddess can be. Bask in her glory, float enraptured on the wings of her joy. *(extended pause—two minutes)*

As the two of you return to yourselves, Ishtar fades from view, and you can feel that she's left a glowing light within you, deep in your core, and you will forever be transformed. If you would like to say anything to the Goddess, do so now, and listen for her answer. *(extended pause—one minute)*

Your lover helps you to your feet and wraps a blanket around you. He bows before you and says, "Gracious and most lovely lady, I will forever remember this day. You have touched and blessed me as the Goddess, and in my heart, so you shall always remain divine."

He has been swept into Ishtar's embrace, and you have been his guide into the realm of the Goddess. As the Sacred Harlot, you have taken him on a journey into the arms of the divine. Think about what this means for you and how this might affect you through the rest of your life. *(extended pause—one minute)*

As he leaves the room, you know that you will never again play the concubine of the Goddess, unless you wish to do so. By submitting your will to the Lady this day, you have learned more about yourself and your ability to be a mirror for the Goddess, to reflect her in your eyes, your heart, your body. *(pause)*

Now let yourself come to rest. Follow my voice. Ten . . . nine . . . you are slowly pulling out of trance. Eight . . . seven . . . six . . . you are becoming awake and aware. Five . . . four . . . you feel your thoughts quickening and stirring. Three . . . two . . . take three deep breaths, and when you awake you will be refreshed and alert. One . . . now take another deep breath, and open your eyes when you are ready.

☾☉☽

After the Meditation

After you have finished the meditation, let yourself drift on the experience for a bit before rising. You might wish to sit with your journal and your fruit and sweets while in bed and write out your thoughts on the ritual. This may affect you in some strong ways. Women are often called sluts and whores when they sleep with someone who isn't their mate, though men are

111

cheered on. Casual sex isn't right for everyone, but it's time for women to reclaim the right to their personal sexuality, time for them to say no or yes based on their true feelings.

We are the face of the Goddess; she's reflected in every woman's eyes, and when we find someone who reveres our sexual self, who sees us in all our beauty and strength, with all our faults and vulnerabilities, the sexual exchange can be charged with a high degree of spiritual energy. We must also learn to acknowledge the divine that exists within the men that we love, and to recognize that they seek union with the Goddess through us, for we are a manifestation of her sacred sex.

When you are ready to open the Circle, take a deep breath and shake out your body. Then face the candle of the Goddess and say:

> *Mighty Ishtar, the Great Har of Babylon, I thank thee for attending this ritual. Go if you must; stay if you will. Leave me blessed and beautiful, understanding my connection to you, to my essence as Woman, through this ritual and rite. Be with me in my heart as I explore the realms of my sex, as I explore what it means to be part of the Goddess, the eternal and divine nature of the feminine. Ishtar, Mother of Civilization, Blessed Be.*

Turn to the west, and say:

> *Spirits of the Water, flow through my life as you lead me into the core of my being, into the hidden depths of my soul, that I might commune with the Divine through my love and my sorrow. Spirits of the Water, thank you for attending this ritual. Farewell, and Blessed Be.*

Turn to the south, and say:

> *Spirits of the Flame, burn in my loins as you pull me into the trance, into the dance, that I might commune with the Divine through my passion and sex. Spirits of the Flame, Farewell and Blessed Be.*

Turn to the east, and say:

Spirits of the Wind, sweep through my body as you remove stagnation and bring a clarity to my spirit, that I might commune with the Divine through spirit and soul and illumination. Spirits of the Wind, Farewell and Blessed Be.

Turn to the north, and say:

Spirits of the Earth, rise up thickly through my feet as you ground me into the energy of my body, that I might commune with the Divine through touch and sense and feeling. Spirits of the Earth, Farewell and Blessed Be.

Now devoke the circle, going widdershins:

I open this Circle, in the name of the Maiden, the Mother, and the Crone, Great Goddess who takes joy in her own body, in her sensuality, in her wit and her wisdom, in her intellect and her play. Be with me throughout the days, Gracious Lady.

Blow out the candle, take another nice bath, and eat a sumptuous meal. Don't try to absorb everything from the ritual in one day; rituals like this can take weeks or even months to fully impact you. Give yourself time.

You may find yourself feeling twinges of guilt if you don't usually fantasize about strangers. This is common, but is a reaction that you should work on. Fantasy about strangers is not unusual, and there is nothing wrong with it. In fact, most fantasies are harmless if kept in the realm of fantasy. Think twice, though, before acting out a fantasy with another person; fantasy's generally best left to the imagination.

Resolve to take more time with your body, exploring your sexuality and your sense of passion for yourself. Learn how to please yourself so you can teach your lover to please you. Don't skimp on finding nonsexual ways to enjoy your body: massage, yoga, movement, long baths, lazing in bed a little more often.

When you think about yourself as a sexual being, remember that you are a mirror of the Goddess in all her facets. She is the Divine Harlot, she is the Embracing Mother, she is the Destroyer, and she is the Creatrix. There will be times when you will want to fuck like a rabbit, and there will be times when you want to make love in a bed of rose petals. Both extremes are valid and are necessary for balance. Listen to which energy you are running on at the time.

Intoxication Oil Version #2

This is one of my favorite and simplest oil blends. No matter what mood I'm in, one whiff can leave me reeling and in a sensuous frame of mind. Blend the following ingredients:

> 40 drops peach oil
> 40 drops dark musk oil
> 5 drops vanilla oil
> 1/4 ounce almond oil

As I said, this is a very simple oil, but the result is incredible. I could sit in a room scented with this for hours.

CHAPTER SIX

Green Men and Stag Kings

Take no scorn to wear the horn
It was the crest when you was born
Your father's father wore it
And your father wore it too.

Hal an tow, jolly rumbelow
We were up long before the day-o
To welcome in the summer,
To welcome in the May-o
The summer is a-coming in
And winter's gone away-o.

"Hal-an-Tow," OLD ENGLISH FOLK SONG

The Stag King represents the Horned God, the Lord of the Forests. He is considered the Goddess's Consort. In many cultures, Celtic society being a prominent example, the king of the land was required to undergo a sacred ritual in which he took on the energy of the Horned God, or Stag King, and joined in sexual union with a priestess representing the Goddess of Sovereignty, or Earth Goddess. Only through the Goddess's acceptance of him in this manner would he be deemed the rightful ruler. As Proinsias Mac Cana says, in *Celtic Mythology:*

> The criterion of a rightful King is that the land should be prosperous and inviolate under his rule—and this can be achieved only if he is accepted as her legitimate spouse by the goddess who personifies his kingdom.

Cernunnos, or Herne, was the Hunter God of the British Isles and is represented by the white stag, as rare and sacred to them as the white buffalo is to Native Americans.

The stag, or King Stag, represents virility, passion, royalty, and lineage, and is often connected with the Wild Hunt. This lord of the forest is also seen in the Green Man and Jack-in-the-Green, whose visages are found across northern Europe as well as in the British Isles. Images of the Green Man usually have vines and leaves twining around the head and sprouting from the mouth, as if the very forest was born from his whisper. Jack-in-the-Green marries the May Queen, Lady of Beltane, and together they bless the fields with their union. The Green Man is life unchecked, insuppressible growth. We see the Green Man's virility in the grass that breaks through concrete streets, in the flowers growing tenaciously in inhospitable places. The King Stag and the Green Man are the undeniable forces of the masculine divine, and you cannot have one without the other. They will not be denied, no matter how much we try to civilize our world. Like the stag's rut or the salmon's drive to spawn upstream, the male principle of fertility and sexuality will be heard.

Most cultures have at least one deity like this—God of the Hunt, God of the Forest and Field, personifying masculine energy. In the Arthurian mythos, the Green Knight serves this purpose, most likely a holdover from the Holly King of the Oak King and Holly King duality. The Finns have Tapio, the Hawaiians have both Lono, God of Agriculture, and Kamapua'a, Vegetation and Pig God.

While most Pagans recognize the idea of the man coming to the Sacred Harlot to partake of the divine, there is a lack of awareness that, throughout history, it has also worked the other way. The woman sometimes went to a representative of the God to partake of the masculine divinity. However, there are differences between the two rituals. Though the Queen of the May is married to the Jack-in-the-Green as a representative of the Goddess, the woman was often seen as a bride for the God. But we find other cases, in more aboriginal cultures, where the girl or woman is definitely seen as a mortal coming to wed the divine god form.

Bêl, a Babylonian god, would choose a mortal woman to stay in his temple, and she would forego intercourse with any mortal man, for she was believed to be the deity's wife. We find a similar situation in Thebes, with the god Ammon. His human wife was known as the Divine Consort, and she was considered to be nearly equal to the queen of Egypt. The queen of Athens was married each year to Dionysus, the god of wine, in a ceremony intended to fertilize the fruit trees and other plants. In India, a Vedic princess was married to the Hindu god Katharagama each summer. Records are unclear as to whether a man represented the god, or whether worshipers used an image made from stone or wood.

The forest and fauna deities are intrinsic parts of Pagan belief and practice. Without the active masculine force, the receptive feminine force cannot quicken. The God fertilizes the Goddess, and from their union, life is born. These gods, above all others, connect with our world in a most primal way. They give us regeneration and the cyclic nature of the seasons. Even the water deities seem more humanized than the forest lords. While the Goddess is eternal, the God is born, brings life and growth, then dies and slides back into the Underworld. We can see this if we look at the Wheel of the Year, with the Goddess being the hub of the wheel, and the God being the rim and spokes that turn around her.

Becoming the Stag King: An Autoerotic Ritual for Men

For your ritual, select the day of a waxing or waning moon depending on whether you want to invoke the God as the Dark Lord (such as Herne or Cernunnos) or as the Bright Lord (such as Pan or Lono). Be sure that you are comfortable touching your own body. If you do not feel comfortable with this, then study chapter 3 and practice those exercises until you can give yourself an orgasm with ease and without guilt.

This ritual is ideally performed outdoors. Just as the women's Sacred Harlot ritual was meant to emulate a temple, so the male's ritual works best in a forest setting. However, realistically, most of you won't have access to a private woodland area. If you can't find an outdoor area where you have complete privacy, then adapt the ritual for the indoor alternative. If you do have private land where you can run around naked, then by all means do so. Just watch out for poison oak and ivy and venomous beasties.

Spend several days preparing for this ritual. Do so in a leisurely fashion; rush nothing during this time. Gather the following items:

- bath salts—patchouli or musk. Find an incense to match, if you like.

- a talisman, an object made from antler, bone, or wood.

- several magazines with images that reflect your idea of sexuality. The day before your ritual, cut sexy, sensual images from these magazines and glue them on a poster board, creating a collage. Hang it in a private space where it can spark your sense of yourself as sexy and vibrant. For more information on creative collage, see my book *Embracing the Moon*.

- fill your room with plants, if you will be indoors, as many as you can. Afterward, you can take care of them or give them away as gifts; you don't want to make the Green Man angry by throwing them away.

a green male-image candle or a phallus-shaped candle, if possible. Otherwise, a green votive or taper candle will do fine. Anoint it with a magical oil like Forest Lord Oil or Woodland Oil. You might also wish to use my Hunting Lord Oil (the recipe follows at the end of this chapter). Anoint the candle with semen.

The day before your ritual, clean your bedroom and arrange to have several hours free from interruption. Tape record the meditation. It's much more effective if you have it on cassette.

On the morning of the ritual, prepare a snack of fruit, meat (if you are not vegetarian), bread, cheese, and wine or grape juice. You might choose beef jerky, apples, cheddar, and port. If you can find wild game, all the better. Do not use alcohol if you are driving to an outdoor area.

The Outdoor Stag King Ritual

Light the incense in your bathroom and set up your collage. Take a leisurely ritual bath with the bath salts. When you are finished, towel off and dress in clothes that you don't mind getting dirty or scuffed, and head for your private spot that you found for your ritual. Take your food, drink, and the talisman.

When you reach your destination and are sure of your privacy, set your food in a safe place. Remove your clothing and, using your talisman, cast a Circle and call on the elements in a manner similar to this:

I cast this Circle once round in the name of the Youth, who takes joy in his own body, who is the face of the Forest Lord unleashed, who runs swiftly through the woodland, leaping tree and branch, splashing in the waters. He is untamed, loving but unpledged, wild and free.

I cast this Circle twice round in the name the Father, who is full in his vigor, who is the face of the God unmatched, who gives and receives from others. It is he who joins with his Lady to mate and to love, to take on the responsibility of the provider and protector.

I cast this Circle thrice round in the name of the Sage, who is the culmination of experience, who is the face of the God wizened and learned. It is he who teaches the arts of the Hunt to those who are new to the chase.

Next invoke the elements. Turn to the north, and say:

Spirits of the Earth, I call thee forth to attend my ritual. Rise up thickly through my feet, you who are the roots of this world, you who are bone and stone and crystal and branch. Ground me into the energy of my body, that I might commune with the Divine through touch and sense and feeling. Spirits of the Earth, manifest in me the Stag King, Forest Lord, that I might wear the antlers that are his crest, that I might express the strength of his body. Welcome, Spirits of the Earth, and Blessed Be.

Turn to the east, and say:

Spirits of the Wind, I call thee forth to attend my ritual. Sweep through my body, you who are mist and vapor, you who are cloud and wind and fog and storm. Remove stagnation and bring a clarity to my spirit, that I might commune with the Divine through spirit and soul and illumination. Spirits of the Wind, manifest in me the Forest Lord, Stag King, that I might wear the vines of his being, so that I might express the clarity of his spirit. Welcome, Spirits of the Wind, and Blessed Be.

Turn to the south, and say:

Spirits of the Flame, I call thee forth to attend my ritual. Burn through my loins, you who are flame and fire, you who are the golden sun, the glowing lava, the rising Phoenix. Pull me into the trance, into the

*dance, that I might commune with the Divine through my passion and
sex. Spirits of the Flame, manifest in me the Forest Lord, Stag King,
that I might wear the fur of his being, so that I might express the
passion of his sexuality. Welcome, Spirits of the Flame, and Blessed Be.*

Turn to the west, and say:

*Spirits of the Water, I call thee forth to attend my ritual. Flow through
my heart and soul, you who are the raging river, the crashing ocean
breakers, the still pool of the grotto. Lead me into the core of my being,
into the hidden depths of my soul, that I might commune with the
Divine through my love and my sorrow. Spirits of the Water, manifest
in me the Forest Lord, Stag King, that I might wear the red eyes of the
Hunter, so that I might express the depths of his emotions. Welcome,
Spirits of the Water, and Blessed Be.*

You will now invoke one of the gods of the Hunt or field. I suggest
Herne, who is less chaotic than Pan or Dionysus. Or you may wish to call
on Lono or Cernunnos. Do a bit of research, and adjust the following invocation appropriately:

*Herne the Hunter! I call to thee. Oh lord of the forest and field, you
who are the Challenger, hear me and join me for this ritual. Invest in
me the feeling of your sacred sexuality, let me understand my connection
to you, to my essence as Man, through this ritual and rite. Be with me,
as I explore the realms of my sex, as I explore what it means to be part
of the God, the cyclic and divine nature of the masculine. Herne, Father
of the Forests, come to me and be with me. Welcome, Gracious Lord,
and Blessed Be.*

When you have invoked the God, take a few moments to feel the touch of
the air on your body, of the sun or breeze as it plays across your skin. At this
point, begin to pleasure yourself. Watch your cock as it becomes erect, feel
your connection to the eternal regenerative force through your maleness.

121

When you are fully aroused, recite next the "Song of Amergin" (see the meditation). With each line, feel your roots to the forest and the earth deepen (see the meditation for visualization suggestions). Call out the words clearly, in a strong voice, and when you are done, take off into the forest. Though you must watch for brambles and poison oak or ivy, your intent is to develop a connection with the strength of the land, to feel yourself rooted in the ground and the trees.

Take time to embrace the trunks of ancient cedars, press yourself close and feel the scratchiness of bark on skin. Roll in the dirt and grass. Fully connect with nature in a playful yet serious way. Every time you touch leaf or branch, know that you are touching an aspect of the Forest Lord. Let your senses, heightened from arousal, lead you into an orgy of making love to the Earth. You are her consort, as the Horned One. You are from her womb, and you are her child, lover, and companion. Maintain your focus as long as possible.

You may find yourself racing through the field laughing, or snuffling in the woods like a boar or stag. Go on all fours for a time. Become the Hunter and become his sacred animals of the Hunt. You are the stag, in rutting season. You are the boar, rooting through the foliage. You are the wolf, watching for rabbits and mice.

When you feel your energy nearing its peak, begin to masturbate and focus your attention on becoming one with the Hunter, on letting your sexuality take you deep into his realm. Sense the passion he has for the Goddess, see her waiting with open arms and open legs for her lover who comes to mate with her. Imagine the joy that he feels when he brings her to orgasm time and again. She is reveling in his touch. She is sexual and wild and passionate; no demure and shy maid this, but the full face of womanhood. And this is what the Hunter wants. She can match him step for step, outpace him, make him struggle to keep up, and the challenge is ever fascinating, ever arousing.

As you bring yourself to a climax, ejaculate on the grass, on the dirt. You are fertilizing the Goddess even as the God does. You are the Hunter incarnate, making love to the Earth.

When you have come back to yourself, slowly return to the place where you left your food and clothing. Sit in the grass naked while you eat, and explore your reactions to the ritual. You might wish to record them. You may have some strong reactions to this ritual. In our culture, men are not encouraged to take pride in their masculinity, but instead are encouraged to be macho, which is a totally different thing. Most men I know are somewhat embarrassed about their bodies, mainly about the way they look naked. The male form hasn't been held up for idealization since the time of the Greeks, except in some areas like bodybuilding. When you are ready to go, devoke the Circle as follows, then dress and return home.

> *Herne the Hunter, Lord of the Forest, I thank thee for attending this ritual. Go if you must, stay if you will. Leave me blessed and glowing, understanding my connection to you, to my essence as Man, through this ritual and rite. Be with me in my heart, as I explore the realms of my sex, as I explore what it means to be part of the God, the eternal and divine nature of the masculine. Herne, Great Challenger, Blessed Be.*

Turn to the west, and say:

> *Spirits of the Water, flow through my life as you lead me into the core of my being, into the hidden depths of my soul, that I might commune with the Divine through my love and my sorrow. Spirits of the Water, thank you for attending this ritual. Farewell and Blessed Be.*

Turn to the south, and say:

> *Spirits of the Flame, burn in my loins as you pull me into the trance, into the dance, that I might commune with the Divine through my passion and sex. Spirits of the Flame, Farewell and Blessed Be.*

Turn to the east, and say:

Spirits of the Wind, sweep through my body, as you remove stagnation and bring a clarity to my spirit, that I might commune with the Divine through spirit and soul and illumination. Spirits of the Wind, Farewell and Blessed Be.

Turn to the north, and say:

Spirits of the Earth, rise up thickly through my feet, as you ground me into the energy of my body, that I might commune with the Divine through touch and sense and feeling. Spirits of the Earth, Farewell and Blessed Be.

Now devoke the Circle, going widdershins:

I open this Circle, in the name of the Young Lord, the Father, and the Sage, Forest Lord who takes joy in his own body, in his sensuality, in his wit and his wisdom, in his intellect and his play. Be with me throughout the days, Gracious Lord.

The Indoor Stag King Ritual

Light the incense in your bedroom and set up your collage and candle. Have the taped meditation and your snack ready. Take a leisurely ritual bath with the bath salts. When you are done, towel dry gently, return to your bedroom, turn on some music, and begin to explore your body. The meditation will come a bit later. First, lull yourself into a sensual trance. Drink a bit of the wine or grape juice and feel it slide down your throat. How does it feel? Is it smooth? Is it fiery?

Cast a Circle and invoke the elements and the God the way you would with the outdoor ritual.

Now lay on your bed or stand in front of your mirror and begin to caress yourself. Run your hands lightly over your body, especially over areas you don't normally think of as sexual. Don't focus on your cock and balls only; explore sensations in your nipples, neck, and other areas.

Sway to the music. Visualize yourself drifting on the wind. Let the music become the breeze and the wind around you. Dance if you wish, for the Lord of Animals is often also the Lord of the Dance. Let yourself go. There is no one here to watch you. As you dance, caress yourself, run your hands over your arms, up and down your legs, through your hair. Lose yourself in the music.

When you are fully aroused, take three deep breaths and let yourself plateau. Settle into this new level of awareness, and turn off the music. Slip your cassette of the meditation in, and lay down on your bed. Follow the words of the meditation as you pleasure yourself. Try to time your orgasm with the pacing in the meditation, but if you can't, don't worry. Just follow the meditation as you drift in an afterglow state.

Meditation for a Stag King Ritual

Take three deep breaths. You are standing in the forest in the late afternoon. The sun filters through the branches of the trees around you, weaving a web of shadow on the ground. Huckleberries and ferns, skunk cabbage, and ancient trees toppled long ago, covered in moss, rest quietly in the droning haze of summer. (pause)

A light breeze plays over your body, and you hear the rustle of the wind through the grass. Or is it a rabbit, a mouse, or a fox? Slowly the heat of the day tugs at your body, loosening the tensions in your muscles, freeing you from thoughts of your daily world and life. There is no rush here, no sense of hurry, and you breathe deeply, free from worry and concern. (pause)

Raise your hands. You find that ivy vines are trailing down from the giant maple trees. Reach out as they coil around your wrists. They slither like snakes, alive and vibrant, aware of your presence. You watch, unafraid, filled with wonder as the ivy writhes onto your body. *(pause)*

A strand of the foliage coils around each of your wrists like a boa, wreathing your arms. Another vine snakes down your torso to coil around your left ankle, and yet another coils around your right ankle. Feel their sleek leaves as they move about your body, embracing you, welcoming you to the forest. *(pause)*

Still another length of ivy coils around your head, creating a wreath of green, a crown of the king. You feel strong here, vibrant and alive. The forest is claiming you for its own. You are melding into the wild. *(pause)*

Take three deep breaths and exhale slowly. *(pause)*

You have come to the forest in search of yourself, in search of union with the Hunter, with he who guards the woodlands. The Lord of Animals, Lord of the Dance, the Green Man. You know him by many names, but the name you know best is Herne. And you seek his blessing today; you seek to join him in a communion with the Divine, in a labyrinth that will lead you back to yourself. *(pause)*

You throw back your head and call out his name three times in a loud, clear voice. "Herne! Herne! Herne!" *(pause)*

After a moment, you feel a rumbling under your feet, and the forest quakes, the earth shakes, and your heart begins to race. From deep in the depths of the woodland, you can feel his presence. From deep in the inner sanctum of his wilderness, you can feel him moving in response to your call. You know who approaches. You know who thunders toward you. Herne, Lord of the Forest. Herne, Lord of the Hunt. Herne, who holds your life in his hands when you walk within his domain. *(pause)*

The very air seems to tremble as the veil of trees parts, and out strides the form of a man, taller than the tallest cedar, broad shouldered with tree-trunk legs and a beard of moss and fur. Atop his crimson-eyed head, you see horns, huge curving antlers that spiral into the sky. As he looks down at you, you notice that he has the biggest erection you've ever seen. *(pause)*

He contemplates your presence for a moment, and then his voice rushes down on a cool blast of wind, whirling around you like a dizzying cacophony of sound. "You have come to my domain, seeking the truth of the Stag King. But to find such a truth, you must first become the stag."

As he speaks, your body begins to shift and, in a painful contortion, you find yourself transforming. Your arms lengthen and your spine stretches. You fall to your hands and knees, arching away from the ground, and as you watch, unable to speak, unable even to moan, your hands and feet shimmer as they change into hooves. *(pause)*

The metamorphosis works its way up your body. Your legs and arms become the legs of the stag; your torso lengthens and thickens. Your cock and balls grow, and you feel them cover over with fur. Then you sense your head shifting, changing into that of a stag, and antlers press through—worrying your head like a new tooth worries a baby's gums—then sprout. *(extended pause—one minute)*

As you transform, Herne begins to recite the "Song of Amergin." With each line, you go deeper into the feeling of truly being the stag. Breathe slowly, deeply, as you listen to his words:

I am a stag: of seven tines,

I am a flood: across a plain,

I am a wind: on a deep lake,

I am a tear: the sun lets fall,

I am a hawk: above the cliff,

I am a thorn: beneath the nail,

I am a wonder: among flowers,

I am a wizard: who but I

Sets the cool head aflame with smoke?

I am a spear: that roars for blood,

I am a salmon: in a pool,

I am a lure: from paradise,

I am a hill: where poets walk,

I am a boar: ruthless and red,

I am a breaker: threatening doom,

I am a tide: that drags to death,

I am an infant: who but I

Peeps from the unhewn dolmen arch?

I am the womb: of every holt,

I am the blaze: on every hill,

I am the queen: of every hive,

I am the shield: for every head,

I am the tomb: of every hope.

As the song builds, you feel a drive in you, a desire to mate. The urge is so strong that you must find a female somewhere. You must find relief. Then, out of the distance, you catch the smell of a female in heat. You are off, racing through tree and bush, so fast that your hooves barely touch the ground. Feel the strength in your legs, the powerful muscles, carrying you forward. The weight of your antlers only seems to add to your virility. Herne follows behind in a cloud of diffused sunlight, as you aim for the object of your desire. *(extended pause—one minute)*

There, in the distance, you see a woman in a diaphanous gown of silk and gauze. She has a full bosom and a round belly, and her eyes are glowing with sparkling light that fills you with a dreadful anticipation. She stands next to a milk-white stag, and you slow to a halt. As you do so, you find yourself taking your own form again, as a man. *(pause)*

She steps forward, and you sense that you are in the presence of no mere mortal, but a goddess. With a laugh, she looks over at Herne, who now stands behind you. "This is your choice for ruler of the realm?" she asks him, and he merely nods.

Ruler? What could she be talking about? But then she looks into your eyes, and you feel her probing, searching your soul. You desire her fiercely, more than you've ever desired any woman before. And you know that if you take her, you will be as a king—respected, royal, honorable. *(pause)*

She puts her hands on your shoulders and gazes into your eyes. Your longing grows. Your cock is erect, and you want to throw her to the ground, to have her fully, but you know that you cannot treat her in this manner. Even if you were so inclined, you sense that she could rip you to shreds without missing a breath.

"Listen to me, and listen well," she says. "To become king of this realm, to walk in the shadow of kings, you must take down the milk-white stag with your bare hands. You must defeat the King to become the King. As it was, so it is, and so it shall always be. The old king will die; the new king will be born. It is a mortal battle of wills—oak and holly, summer and winter, new and old. The winner will mate with me to claim his rightful throne." *(pause)*

In her words, you see the cycle, the turning of seasons, life and death and then life again. Eternally spinning, this wheel has turned since the beginning of time and shall continue to turn long after you are gone. This is your time in the hub. Here is your chance to swing upwards on the turn of the spokes. You see the cycling of life. The silverback ages and is dethroned by the younger gorillas, the old bull wearies and is gored by the young ones; all over the world, all over the lands, this drama plays itself out. And now it is your time to rise. *(extended pause—two minutes)*

She backs away, and the white stag moves forward. He is ancient. You can sense the weight of the years on his shoulders, and as he looks at you, you can see his desire to rest. But he cannot step aside. According to the cycle, he must be defeated. You cautiously move in, circling, wary of the antlers that rise, threatening and sharp. *(pause)*

He snorts, paws the ground, lowers his head. You jostle for a position in back of him, where he cannot get at you. He bellows and charges forward, and you leap to the side just in time to avoid being gored. As you do, you swiftly turn and lunge for his neck, embracing him as you make contact. *(pause)*

The stag tries to throw you, but you hold tight, scrambling for purchase against his ancient body. You can feel Herne watching you, and you remember the strength that you felt when you raced as the stag. Call that strength back into your body now. It will give you power. Remember the movements; remember the vitality. *(pause)*

The battle intensifies. The stag manages to flip his head back and scratch you with one antler tip. A line of blood glistens on your torso. But you hold fast though you realize he is deadly serious. The King Stag will kill you if he can, for his honor and the cycle demand a sacrifice. You take a deep breath and throw yourself against him. The power of the stag in your body gives you the energy to take him down to the ground. *(extended pause—one minute)*

Now the white stag is enraged, and he thrashes wildly, lashing out with hooves and horns. He lands a blow on your chest; it knocks you back, but you lunge again and this time you catch hold of his antlers. You have him now. One good twist with the adrenaline and divine energy flowing through your body, and you will break his neck. You gaze into his eyes, sorrow filling your heart that you have to kill this creature, but you see in his returning look that he did the same when he was young, as did his opponent before him, and so on back through time immemorial. *(pause)*

Herne leans forward, and you hear the thunder of his words. "You are the Hunter. Never let your prey suffer; never inflict more pain than you have to." And you know the time is now. You must do this deed, and you must do it quickly. With one quick twist, you hear the sound of crunching bones, and the stag convulses and goes limp. *(extended pause—one minute)*

Even as tears cascade down your cheeks, you hear a cry ring out. "The king is dead! Long live the king!" As you turn, the forest is alive with animals of all kinds, and wood spirits and the energy from every tree and shrub surround you. *(pause)*

The woman walks up to you and offers her hand. "You have but one task left, Hunter, before you can be declared King. Come and join with me."

She slips out of her dress, letting it fall to the ground, and stands regal, naked, with flowing hair and brilliant eyes. "Do you know who I am?" she asks, and her question demands an answer.

You nod, for you now know who you are facing. "You are the Goddess of Sovereignty," you say. She smiles. She is Queen of the Land. She is the land, and only those with whom she mates may claim the right to rule as King. She is law and justice, she is the Earth Mother incarnate. She wears many faces and many names, but every aspect of her being claims the right to choose those who rule this world. *(pause)*

And now she leads you to a field, where the furrows have been ploughed and seeds planted but nothing yet grows. "Touch me, quicken me; make bountiful that which is fallow with your seed."

You reach out and slide your hand over her breast and feel the nipple stiffen. The heady scent of her sex drifts up, and you find yourself hard, erect, and aching. But she is Queen of the Land, and you must pay your respects. Beginning at her feet, you move your lips up her body—up her ankle, ringing it with kisses, then along her calf to the back of her knee. With your hand, you stroke her other leg, her skin soft under your fingers. She moans slightly and parts her legs just enough for you to slip your hand between them. *(pause)*

A light breeze drifts by as you continue your kisses—up the back of her thighs, to her buttocks, where you gently bite the plump, round flesh. She shifts her hips, and you slide your hand up the inside of her thighs. Then she reaches down, takes your hand, and pulls you up to face her. Her lips meet yours, and she probes your mouth with her tongue. *(pause)*

You feel one of her hands slip down to cup your balls; she gently strokes them, then squeezes just enough to send a thrill up your spine. You want her now, but you know that if you wait, she will give you even more pleasure than you thought possible. She drags you to the ground, and her desire excites you more. As she leans back, you take one of her breasts in your mouth, tonguing the nipple, sucking hard as she moans. With one hand, you stroke her hair; with the other, you reach down and slide your fingers into her cunt, which is slick and hot. *(pause)*

After a moment, she pushes you back, then grins and turns, slipping over your body so her head is near your cock. You are staring up into her womanhood, and you can see the swollen button, the glistening lips that await your mouth. As you pull on her hips to bring her closer so your tongue can explore her depths, you feel her moist, warm tongue as she takes your cock in her mouth and begins to suck. *(pause)*

Your already stiff member becomes tighter as you feel her lips close around you, sliding down the shaft, licking, swirling over the swollen glans. She moans as she milks you, biting so gently you can barely feel her teeth. As you tongue-bathe her, she stiffens, cries out, and you can feel the contractions of orgasm sweep through her body. A surge of your own tells you that your orgasm is near, but you don't want to come yet; you don't want it to be over that soon. *(pause)*

With a swift twist, you roll her over, underneath you, and she spreads her legs. One thrust, and you're inside of her—deep, pushing all the way to the back. She's so moist that it feels like you're in the middle of the ocean, waves rocking the two of you from side to side. You drive into her again and again, alternating slow, steady strokes with short, quick bursts. She smiles, crying out your name, and you see the radiance of the divine surrounding her, even as you feel the power of Herne rushing through your body. The rhythm builds, the tempo quickens, and there is a brilliant flash as you let go thought, let go of control, and climax. *(extend pause— two minutes)*

As you return to yourself, the Goddess separates from you and gives you a gentle kiss. "I proclaim you the King of the land. You are the rightful ruler of this domain and all that walk within. You answer to myself and Herne alone in this world."

As you rise and turn, Herne laughs and says, "Now you know the power of the Stag. Now you know the power of the Hunter, and the responsibility. You are ready now to meet the challenges that I may present to you."

If you have anything you would like to say or ask of him at this time, then do so now, and listen for his answer. *(extended pause— one minute)*

Now let yourself come to rest. Follow my voice. Ten . . . nine . . . you are slowly pulling out of trance. Eight . . . seven . . . six . . . you are becoming awake and aware. Five . . . four . . . you feel your thoughts quickening and stirring. Three . . . two . . . take three deep breaths, and when you awake you will be refreshed and alert. One . . . now take another deep breath, and open your eyes when you are ready.

After the Meditation

After you have finished the meditation, let yourself drift on the experience for a bit before rising. You might wish to sit with your journal and your meat and bread while in bed and write out your thoughts on the ritual. This may affect you in some strong ways. The ritual killing of the stag may present you with difficulties if you have a gentle nature, but remember, if you eat meat, it was once a live animal and had to be slaughtered for your consumption. If you are a vegetarian, you destroy life from the earth to survive with every salad, every bite of carrot or grain. We must face the cycle and not be afraid of it, while respecting all that walk its path.

You are the face of the God; he is reflected in every man's eyes, and when you find someone who reveres your sexual aspect, who sees you in all your strength and vigor, with all your faults and vulnerabilities, the sexual exchange can be charged with a high degree of spiritual energy. You must learn also to see the divine within the women that you care for, and to recognize that women seek union with the God through you, for you are a manifestation of his sacred sex.

When you are ready, open the Circle as directed in the section for the outdoor ritual, take a deep breath, and shake out your body. Blow out your candle, take another bath, and eat a hearty meal. Don't try to absorb everything from the ritual in one day. Rituals like this can take weeks or even months to fully impact you. Give yourself time.

Follow the ritual with a camping trip with male friends who understand this type of energy, who won't get caught up in locker-room games and stories. Plan an all-male ritual to explore the sides of yourselves that you keep locked away for fear of ridicule. This includes not only your sensitivities, but your fears about your own sexuality.

Sometimes in Paganism, we lessen the importance of male divinity, a response to the overwhelming patriarchy that has held sway for so long. While understanding the cause of this, we can begin to change these attitudes by focusing on positive masculine attributes, which include strength and vigor and sexuality and even competition and aggression (all of these are human qualities, really, rather than just masculine traits), and by leaving behind the good ol' boys' network that still seems rampant among a number of wannabe Vikings (I'm not talking about true Norse Paganism here, a totally different matter) and the "I-am-man-hear-me-roar" attitudes that sometimes come out of many men's groups.

Next time you eat a steak dinner, or chicken, or any other type of animal, remember where it came from, think about the food chain and the cycle. Thank the creature for its life, for without the Hunter, a lord of death as well as life, we would not have these foods to eat.

Hunting Lord Oil

This oil can be used whenever you wish to invoke the power of the Forest Lord. See my book, *Embracing the Moon,* for instructions on how to raise energy and charge the oils.

> 12 drops patchouli oil
> 10 drops cedar oil
> 10 drops musk oil
> 8 drops vetiver oil
> 2 drops rose oil
> 2 drops lemon oil
> $1/4$ ounce almond oil

Blend, charge, and store in a dark bottle out of the sunlight.

CHAPTER SEVEN

Sex and Magic:
Divine Communion

This is the very ecstasy of love.

WILLIAM SHAKESPEARE, *Hamlet*

I will not be talking about or teaching Eastern tantric techniques here. Eastern tantra, or tantra yoga, is a strict discipline and should only be practiced by those who have devoted years to the study. While sexuality is a major part of Eastern tantra, it is not the goal, nor is the goal in Eastern tantra simply to reach the divine through sexuality. Instead, I will be leading you on a somewhat different journey.

The last few chapters were devoted to exploring sexual communion with the divine on a solitary basis; this chapter is geared to couples who wish to practice sex magic and sexual communion together. I focus on heterosexual couples, but same-sex couples can alter the information as they need to; most of the exercises are easily practiced by people of any persuasion.

The most important thing for a couple to remember is that the goal is to be comfortable together. Sexuality is a personal experience, and it's vital that each couple tailors rituals to their specific needs as a couple and their needs as individuals.

We will explore three aspects of sacred sexuality in a couples situation:

- ⥥ communing with the divine through sexual intercourse

- ⥥ learning how to use the energy of that sexual connection for spell-work and magic

- ⥥ exploring the Great Rite or the Hieros Gamos—the divine union or Sacred Marriage (in chapter 8)

Acknowledging Your Partner's Divine Nature

To commune with the divine through sexual play with another, you must first be able to see divinity within your partner, to look in their eyes and see the face of the God or Goddess. This requires that you respect your partner. Too often partners take one another for granted, losing track of that which drew them together in the first place.

When you marry or partner with someone, you do so because of the qualities you see in them at that time, not just for future potential. Don't expect your partner to suddenly change their nature because you're married. If she is sexy and passionate and lives life with a zest, don't expect her to suddenly become sedate and content with staying home every evening. Revel in the fact that she's a sexual and passionate woman who happens to love you.

When you fall in love with a man's fun-loving and free spirit, don't expect him to sell his bike and buy a station wagon the moment you move in together. Give him room to be that freewheeling man who captured your heart in the first place. Let him remain a little wild.

This is not to say that we should stand in the way of positive change. However, a person can only change when they are ready to and want to. Contrary to what grandma used to say, love alone won't produce miracle transformations; if you expect your partner to drastically alter his or her behavior just because you fall in love, you're going to be disappointed.

What first drew you to your mate? Remember the qualities that you loved about them when you first met. Love will deepen and change; you both will mature and go through transitions. You can't force a change if it's not the right time and you can't make someone over into the image of who you think they should be.

To evolve, we must undergo periodic transformation or stagnation sets in, and from there discontent. We need to find a balance that allows us the space to grow yet keeps our relationship alive. We must respect the changes in each other as we learn and grow from our experiences, and we must not exclude our partners as we evolve.

Sound complicated? It is.

A committed, one-on-one relationship seems like a recipe for insanity. Take two individuals and attempt to create a unified life for them together. Stir well to blend while retaining a sense of autonomy and personal freedom. It's like making a checkerboard cake—take chocolate and vanilla batters and figure out how to pour them into the same pan and create a unified whole without blending the flavors into one unidentifiable mess. It can be done, but it requires communication, honesty, and flexibility.

Too often, people feel that they should give up their individuality within a relationship. If you give up who you are, what's left?

When you unite with another person, you are essentially creating a union of three people—you, me, and us. This requires respect and compromise. I see people who treat their partners worse than they treat their pets or belongings. A good gauge to use when you're in a difficult period is to stop and ask yourself, "Would I treat my best friend the way I'm treating my partner?" If the answer is, "No, I'd never say something that cruel to my best friend!" or "I'd never leave my dog alone for a week and expect him to be happy about it!" then perhaps you need to reevaluate how you relate to your lover.

I'm not talking about play, where you both fully understand that you're joking. Samwise jokes about how bitchy I am, and I joke about how forgetful he is. While there is truth behind the humor, we don't let our irritation become a weapon, and we both fully acknowledge our faults. Rather, I'm talking about sarcastic jabs and prods where you may say, "Oh, I'm just teasing," but you can see the hurt in your partner's eye. Or nights where you stay out with your friends and conveniently "forget" to let your mate know when to expect you.

If you find yourself becoming physically violent, you have a serious problem and you need to find help immediately. You have no right to expect your mate to take such abuse. Unfortunately, an abused partner often stays out of fear, insecurity, or low self-esteem, but I guarantee you from experience they aren't staying because they like that sort of treatment and they aren't staying out of true love. The mantra of any relationship should be: There is no excuse for abuse.

I've said it before, and I'll say it again: *If you find yourself in an abusive relationship, get out now.* Forget the family china, forget the house, forget Auntie Ivy's hand-carved armoire. Your life comes first. People actually die from daily abuse. Women and men alike can find themselves victims of domestic abuse. Abuse crosses gender preference lines, cropping up in homosexual as well as heterosexual relationships. Do you want your children to grow up and learn that abuse is a normal part of a relationship? Stay in a bad situation and that's exactly what will happen.

Don't expect things to get better miraculously. I'm sorry, but they won't. I speak from experience. I spent almost nine years of my life waiting for things to "get better." When someone keeps saying "I'm sorry, it won't happen again," it's part of the cycle of abuse and will not end without professional help. Take your kids, if you have any, get the hell out, and seek help. You may be saving your life, and you will certainly be saving your sanity.

Respect for your partner includes encouraging them to grow intellectually and spiritually, even if they grow in a different direction from you. One of the best ways to develop mutual support is to respect yourself. If you're secure about yourself, you'll be comfortable celebrating your mate's successes. You'll be strong enough to cushion them when they need your reassurance. If you sneer at their hopes and goals, what kind of partner are you? And if you ignore your responsibility in a marriage or partnership, what does that say about your respect for your mate?

This works both ways. For a relationship to work, to grow and flourish, both partners must accept responsibility and uphold whatever vows were made.

You must also respect your mate's right to privacy. Indeed, if you are using this book together as a guide, then recognize that you both need alone time to explore your individual sexuality. You will become better partners if your sex life together is healthy. Let your lover teach you what they learn about their own responses. You can then increase their pleasure when you're making love. Learn to communicate about what you want from sex. This is vital to a successful relationship.

The right to privacy also includes staying out of her purse and keeping out of his wallet, unless you have permission. Everyone needs a space to call their own, even if it's a small one. Do you trust your partner? Do they respect your vows? Then don't be threatened by their desire for a little privacy.

Your mate is your partner, not your possession. Sam stays out of my office unless he knocks first, or if I'm in another room and he really needs to get something. We don't read each other's email. When I go out with male friends, he doesn't prod me to find out where we went and what we did; I've been gone all day and evening with my guy friends before, and he's never jumped to erroneous conclusions. When he gives women at his workplace rides home, I don't automatically freak out and accuse him of cheating on me.

When you respect your partner, when you look upon them as a face of the God or Goddess, then it is possible to develop a deep spiritual connection with them.

One of the exercises I've led in workshops runs this way: turn to the person and look directly into their eyes. Then give them a compliment. They must not whisk it away or negate it, but accept it with a heartfelt and simple, "Thank you." Then they will turn to you and do the same. You can practice this exercise with your partner on a daily basis. This develops a sense of reverence between you and increases self-esteem.

Setting Up an Altar and Invocations to the Gods

You might wish to set up a sex altar in your bedroom. You can use any colors that have special significance for you, but red is the traditional color of passion. Red or fuchsia and black makes an erotic color scheme, but match it to your bedroom color theme so it isn't discordant. Set up the altar on your dresser or on a shelf or table where it won't be disturbed.

Find a cloth that you like. One of the easiest ways to obtain altar cloths is at a fabric store; you don't have to hem the cloth if you don't want to, although it can prevent snags and runs.

I suggest finding a source for sex candles. Use yoni-shaped ones for women and phallic ones for men. If your nearest witchcraft shop doesn't have them, there are plenty of online and mail-order shopping sites for magical supplies. You may wish to carve runes or words like "sacred sex," "passion," or "magnetic attraction," on your candles. Men should anoint their cock candles with seminal fluid; women should anoint their yoni candles with vaginal juices. I also recommend anointing a candle with an oil like Lovers Oil (the recipe is given on page 146) or my Nymph & Satyr Oil (which is found in my book *Embracing the Moon*).

Place the candles so they are almost touching in a pretty, heat-proof receptacle half-filled with salt, and set them on your altar cloth. If you can't find yoni- and lingam-shaped candles, image candles or standard taper or votive candles will work.

You may wish to add a picture of yourselves to the altar if you are married or handfasted, along with your handfasting cord, flowers, and gemstones. Perhaps you would like a statue of Shakti and Shiva, Aphrodite and Pan, or other deities related to sex. When you are exploring sex magic, if you choose to cast a Circle, you can call the elements and light your candles. This creates a sense of tradition and unity and can heighten your experience together. During your rites, you might wish to invoke deities for your sexual exercises and rituals. Sample invocations to Shiva and Shakti follow.

Invocations to Shiva and Shakti

During late 1998, I began to feel drawn to Eastern philosophy. I resisted, afraid that if I dove in, I might not come up. I finally had to accept that this was a study and path I needed to walk for a while. I explored the concept of the Tao. Writing poetry focused on transcending while still in the body, I began connecting with Shiva and Shakti. In 1999, during the research and planning for this book, the pull to the East grew stronger, and I found myself hungry for information on Hinduism, longing to see the sacred temples in India.

A few months before Sam and I started invoking Shakti and Shiva into our sex magic, I had a dream. I dreamed of a blue god, striding across the land toward me, weapons in all four of his hands. Petrified, I knew that if he reached me, he would kill me in a death more terrifying than any I had ever imagined. I frantically tried to slice my wrists, hoping to die before he could touch me. I realize now that this dream was the manifestation of my fears about transformation, about writing *Crafting the Body Divine* and *Sexual Ecstasy & the Divine*, about how these books would leave my life forever changed. It was also an indication that Shiva was watching and waiting.

The first time Sam and I invoked Shakti and Shiva into our rites, I actually saw Shiva standing behind Samwise; just a glimpse, but the Blue God was there. Another time, after our invocations, I felt a strong sense of Shakti filtering through my body. When I looked at Samwise, he said, "You look different; your face just changed." I knew the divine pair were with us again.

Shiva, Lord of Compassion, Lord of Yogis, Triple-Eyed God, Prince of Demons, hear me. Blue God, you who wield the trident, you who are Lord of the Dance, come to me. Lord of opposites, you who are god of purity, you who are lord of outcastes. Shiva, master of asceticism, lord of passion, be with me in my rites, in my body, in my life as I explore the divine connection between you and your consort Shakti, without whom you cannot act, with whom you are eternally bound.

Shakti, Great Mother of the Universe, you whose dance awakens your Lord Shiva, hear me. Lady of creation, crone of destruction, within you blossoms the compassion and beauty of Parvati, within you burn the fires of Kali-Ma. Shakti, keeper of the sacred lotus, be with me in my rites, in my body, in my life as I explore the divine connection between you and your consort Shiva, without whom you cannot act, with whom you are eternally bound.

Lovers Oil

This oil is very powerful. Make sure you use it around those you want to be attractive to. Blend well, charge with energy, and store in a dark bottle.

> $^1/_2$ ounce almond oil
> 25 drops rose oil
> 25 drops lotus oil
> 10 drops jasmine oil
> 10 drops ylang-ylang oil

10 drops sandalwood oil

flowers: rose or jasmine

gem: turquoise or garnet

Sensuous Breath Control

Just as you must exercise your body to become adept physically, and your mind to become adept intellectually, so you must practice sexual exercises to heighten your experiences with sexual communion and sex magic. Controlling your breath can elevate sexual responses.

When you are starting to get aroused but before you begin sex play in earnest, take three slow deep breaths. Focus on the sensations running through your body. Work through your muscles, slowly tensing each one, then letting it relax. Breathe slowly as you go; don't hyperventilate. Your goal is to prepare your body for the buildup of energy. Throughout all your sexual play, alone or with partners, you can use breath control to channel and increase your pleasure.

Breathe in a full and rhythmic manner. Short, shallow breaths will tighten your muscles and distract your focus from the sexual tension. Lack of oxygen prevents blood from flowing freely through your veins. Breathe from your diaphragm, slowly. Cycle your breath in a circle—in through your nose, down your windpipe, into your lungs. Feel it travel through your bloodstream, through your body, then bring it back up again and exhale through your mouth. Eventually, this will become a habit, and you won't have to think about it.

During a highly aroused state, it may be difficult to remember to breathe in this manner, but the more you do so, the more you will enjoy sex. Rhythmic breathing can also help you fall into trance, which is conducive to the exercises and rituals here and to all of your magical practice.

Exchanging Breath: The Sacred Kiss

There are kisses and then there are kisses. Expert sexologists recommend that couples practice deep kissing at least once a day. I'm not talking about a peck on the cheek, but a full-scale, ten-second-long, tongue-tasting kiss. Here, we take this a step further.

The sacred kiss is an exchange of energy and breath between partners. You can either stand or lay down for this; whichever you choose, try to have full body contact. Stare into each other's eyes for this exercise. Begin by taking a full breath, and then kiss. You will need to time this at first, to get the idea of how long a full minute is when you are kissing without a break. You might want to set a timer that doesn't have a loud buzzer to guide you.

Visualize your energy running in a circle, from your Kundalini up your spine. Instead of allowing it to pass out through your crown chakra, focus it into your mouth and through your lips into your partner's mouth. They should do the same with their energy. When you breathe in, pull their energy into you and run it down through your spine. Cycle it down through your spine into your genitals, where it can blend with your own Kundalini force.

During sexual intercourse, you and your partner may use this exercise to blend and cycle your energies, then draw on that blended energy through genital contact. When both genitals and lips are touching, you have two complete cycles of energy running simultaneously—from you into your partner and from your partner into you.

When you orgasm, release this energy out of your crown chakra to connect with the universal force. If you are not going to continue from the kiss into sexual intercourse, then you should release the energy in some other manner, either through exercise or masturbation.

Nonsexual Erotic Touching

Nonsexual erotic touching is common to many sexual practices, both spiritual and nonspiritual, and is often used when sexual dysfunction crops up in a relationship. It helps the partners become comfortable with one another again and takes some of the pressure of "performance" off the couple. You're going to use it to heighten the awareness of your body, your partner's body, and how your partner reacts to your touch.

You will need a clock or watch or hourglass for this exercise. Both partners should be nude. Make sure the room is at a comfortable temperature and that you are both feeling good. If you approach this exercise when you are in a bad mood or when you are ill or tired, you aren't likely to have a good experience. An imaginary couple, Paul and Mary, will demonstrate the next two exercises.

Have one person lay down on the bed. Our couple decides that Paul will go first. He lays down on his stomach. For five minutes, Mary runs her hands all over his back, into every crease, though avoiding the anal area (which is considered an erogenous zone). She can trail her hair over him, rub her breasts across his skin, use her feet—anything to produce pleasant sensations. When her five minutes are up, the couple switches places, with Mary on her stomach, and Paul doing the same to her. They do this twice.

Next, Paul turns on his back, and Mary again touches him all over, avoiding his genitals and nipples. Five minutes later, they switch places. They repeat the exercise. If a partner is aroused at this point, the couple can go on to have sex, or they can stop for the evening, but neither partner should feel obligated to have sex if they don't want to. If Mary is aroused but Paul is too tired for sex, he can hold her in his arms while she masturbates, or he can masturbate her to orgasm.

Sexual Erotic Touching

Follow the preceding instructions for nonsexual erotic touching. Now begin a session of sexual erotic touching.

Paul is again on his stomach; this time Mary begins to touch him erotically, running her hands between his legs to finger his scrotum, lightly caressing his anus, kissing his buttocks, licking his spine. After five minutes, they switch places. Then they repeat the exercise.

Paul next turns onto his back, and Mary caresses him all over, including his cock and balls, his nipples. During this phase, she can use her hair, her tongue, her lips, or her fingers to sexually arouse her partner. She doesn't focus on the genitals, but includes them in her play. After five minutes, Mary lays on her back to receive Paul's attentions. They do this a second time.

At this point, you'll probably be aroused, and you should either masturbate each other to orgasm or make love. Do not rush your sexual play. Too often, this is the time when women experience disappointment. While foreplay is wonderful, intercourse is often hurried and rushed. Take your time.

Both of these exercises will heighten your sensitivity to touch; they include the whole body and can break down inhibitions about specific body parts. With erotic touching, we sanctify the whole body. Every part of you is sacred and loveable. Every nook and cranny holds hidden delights. When we fully learn our partner's body by touch, we develop a stronger bond on both physical and emotional levels. By mingling our auras through this practice, we become attuned to each other's energy on a deeper level.

The Art of Thrusting

One of the problems a number of men have is lasting long enough for the woman during actual intercourse. This technique will help prolong an erection and is very pleasurable for most women. It also allows the couple time to reach a meditative state during intercourse, which will help in the quest for divine communion. One of the easiest ways to practice the art of thrusting is from the rear-entry position, where the man kneels behind the woman who is on her hands and knees. If her arm muscles or wrists are weak, she can lay across some propped-up pillows.

The man should begin with shallow strokes. You might want to establish a rhythm, perhaps seven shallow strokes where the penis just barely enters the vagina. Aim for penetrating no more than the length of the glans, or head of your cock, then pull out and enter again. Do not pull out all the way, but just to the tip of your penis. Shallow thrusts should be done quickly. This will build up excitement in the woman and make her hungry for more. Then shift to long, deep thrusts, done slowly. Again, keep to a rhythm, perhaps seven shallow, four deep. Experiment; vary the tempo. The longer, deeper thrusts will make her feel satiated and full. The variation in rhythm helps him prolong his erection and avoid premature ejaculation.

Same-sex couples can adjust this exercise to suit their preference. Lesbians can use a dildo to simulate the penis, while queers can work with either anal sex or an oral variation.

Women take note: Sexual thrusting (and reaching orgasm through intercourse) helps ease menstrual cramps. A vibrator can also help, but the thrusting is more effective.

Plateaus and Pleasure

Thrusting speed needs to be addressed, too. Men tend to thrust quickly during sex, while women respond to a slow buildup, followed by a faster conclusion. Whatever you prefer, the pleasures of plateaus can enhance a sexual relationship.

Allowing yourselves to plateau together is one of the quickest ways I've found to heighten your sexual energy and passion. During sex, when you are starting to near orgasm, stop all movement, but stay joined. Breathe

151

deeply, but keep your thoughts focused on the sensations of how your partner feels under your touch. Don't let the energy slip away. Acclimate yourself to this new level of heightened passion. When you finally orgasm, your climax will be even greater.

They are near orgasm, hot for each other, passionate and in love. He thrusts deep within her, driving her nearer and nearer the edge. She holds up her hand and motions for him to be still. He stops, cock so deep inside her that it feels like she's impaled on his scepter. They pause, silent, focusing on the energy passing between them.

They breathe deeply, slowly, allowing the heat to build again. Their skin is on fire; the feel of his cock begins to drive her wild. She can't stay still much longer, and yet she does, focusing on the ache, the hunger to move. Finally, with the air charged and glowing around them, he begins to move again, short shallow strokes, deep penetrating thrusts, and she returns his motions, squirming under his relentless exploration of her inner gardens. Once again, she motions for him to stop, and he waits. Again they let the passion build further.

With each plateau, they acclimate to a heightened state of awareness. She can almost feel herself inside his body now. He can feel himself looking through her eyes. And then, finally, they race for the summit, entwining, grinding together in an ecstasy of motion, a blur of two bodies joined. As she comes, he can feel her reach for the Gods and meet them. As he orgasms, she feels herself rising up with him, ascending to the realm of the Gods. They are communing not only with the Divine, but with one another.

Slowly, they return to their bodies, to their separate selves, joined and yet once again individual. Their bond is tighter; their love a little stronger. The fire has been stoked again, and they feed it with their passion.

There have been times when I have actually been in my own body and felt myself inside Samwise's aura, his energy, as he climaxed. Bilocation, to a degree. This doesn't happen all that often, but when it does I am so connected to him that I am no longer myself; I am a part of the sexual dance that creates the universe.

Sex at this level can be all-encompassing and involves a passion that goes beyond the body and merges the partners into a union that is both expansive and exclusive. Macrocosm and microcosm. When you touch the Divine in your partner, you touch the Divine in the universe.

We discussed plateaus in chapter 3, where I used the analogy of climbing a set of stairs. If you stop to rest several times, while maintaining your focus, you will make it much farther up the staircase than you would have otherwise. This takes practice and may require several sessions before you are familiar enough with the signs indicating how close you are to orgasm. But as always, the journey is delicious, and the process is a key to enlightenment.

Orgasm without Ejaculation

This is an interesting topic, and I'm not sure how I feel about it. I am female, so I can't speak from firsthand experience. Samwise does not practice this, but I've talked to some men who do. Opinions have varied from "wonderful" to "it's okay now and then." What it boils down to is learning to control your sexual functions so you can orgasm one or more times without ejaculating. Eastern philosophies maintain that this preserves the man's vital essence. Indeed, some tantric adepts have been known to ejaculate into the woman; then use their penis much like a straw to suck up the ejaculate along with her fluids.

In many of these philosophies, the woman is seen as having an inexhaustible supply of sexual energy, but the man's supply is seen as limited, so he must retain what he can and renew himself with the woman's sexual energy.

I have met some men who are multiorgasmic (a trait more often associated with women than men). However, most of these men ejaculate. But they have learned how to have several orgasms before they do. If we accept the commonly held theory that the brain is the biggest sex organ and that a lot of our sexuality resides in our attitude, then we can see how men can become multiorgasmic through use of visualization, attitude, and a heightened sensual self (without having to learn a long and complicated Eastern process). If you don't have the time or a teacher, you can simulate some aspects of multiorgasm through a different approach. The erotic touching exercises will help, and so will practicing your Kegel exercises to strengthen your PC muscles. (A reminder, both men and women should practice their Kegel exercises daily.)

If you would like to explore nonejaculatory orgasm, read *Passion Play* by Felice Dunas and *The Art of Sexual Ecstasy* by Margo Anand. They will get you started and point the way to other texts that will help.

Orgasms: Am I Having One?

Men have an obvious reaction that signals their orgasms—they ejaculate. Some men, as we discussed, can learn to be multiorgasmic. For women, however, it's not so cut-and-dried. It took me years to have an orgasm after I started having sex.

So much of the process is cerebral that I believe many blocks to achieving a climax are psychological—not understanding how orgasm works, not understanding that it's different for each woman, being out of touch with your body, being so uptight about your looks that you block pleasure, and being with inept lovers.

If you are having difficulty achieving orgasm, I recommend that you practice masturbation. It's much easier to focus on your reactions when you are alone, and this will allow you the freedom you need to discover what works best for you. You might find that you were so worried about your partner's pleasure that you were ignoring your own signals. You might discover that you need more buildup to orgasm; five minutes of foreplay isn't enough for any woman when they're starting cold, from a nonaroused state. If you are embarrassed about your lack of experience, you may freeze up. Illness and fatigue are also vital factors in an inability to achieve a climax.

Orgasm is a physical release of energy that affects your entire body. Most often, the strength of this release will depend on a number of factors. You may find at times that you are stunned—shrieking or laughing or crying as a cascade of energy rushes through your body. Other times, it may be quick, sort of a whoosh, and then it's gone. Or you may feel a flush and a quick jolt and boom, then back to earth again. All of these experiences are legitimate; all of them are orgasmic. Don't expect every time to be like you see in the movies, with screaming and total passionate surrender. It's not always like that, and that's okay. Explaining orgasm is a little like explaining the way a sneeze feels; in fact, the two processes are rather similar. Sometimes it's a little "achoo," and other times it's a huge explosion.

Masturbation will help you divine your body's responses. Get to know how your orgasms work. We must take responsibility for our own sexuality. How can we expect our partners to know how to bring us to orgasm if we can't achieve the same thing ourselves?

If you don't think you have had an orgasm, well, you probably haven't. If you continue to have difficulties, talk to your gynecologist to see whether there is a medical reason for your lack of arousal.

Positions, Positions, Which Position?

There are so many choices, aren't there? Actually, that's not entirely true. There are many variations of a few basic positions. Some books give interesting names (most derived from the Kama Sutra) for each variation. I'm going to avoid romanticism and mysticism here for the sake of clarity.

The most basic positions are: face-to-face, man on top (missionary); face-to-face, woman on top; rear entry (man behind woman); standing; and seated (woman on man's lap). Within these parameters lies an infinite variety of possibilities.

Missionary. So named as the position that the missionaries felt was most righteous. They tried to instill this as the only acceptable position when they invaded and converted native cultures. In this position, the man kneels between the woman's thighs as she lays on her back. He enters her from this position, and she may either keep her knees bent or wrap her legs around him, or he can put her legs up over his shoulders as he kneels and enters her. This position promotes the most eye contact and is best when the man isn't too much heavier than the woman and the woman isn't very large. The missionary position is among the least favorites, coming in behind woman on top and rear entry in most polls.

Woman on top. This is a perennial favorite. The woman straddles the man, either facing his chest or turned so she is facing his legs. This position allows the woman more freedom of movement and takes some of the pressure off the man to perform. Women of all sizes can use this position, which allows partners who are disparate in size to enjoy passionate contact without having to figure out challenging logistics (for example, he is six-four and she is five-two, or he is 150 pounds and she is 250 pounds). Contrary to your fears, ladies, you will not squash your partner even if he's smaller than you; your knees on either side of his body support most of your weight. Men enjoy this position because it allows them to look up at their partner's breasts and face, and it makes it easier to stimulate her clit during intercourse.

Rear entry. Often called "doggie style," the most common variation of this position is with the woman kneeling on her hands and knees. The man kneels behind her and inserts his cock into her vagina from this angle. Rear entry allows for the deepest thrusting of the man into the woman, and it is more feral than other positions. Some people see this position as "dirty" or "racy" and often women don't realize that it's not the same thing as anal intercourse and so are afraid to try it. Other variations of the rear entry position are with the woman leaning down with her breasts touching the floor, or with the man standing at the end of the bed as the woman kneels on the edge. The rear-entry position is especially good for a woman who is large-sized or pregnant, or a man who really likes to be able to grab hold of his partner's hips so he can thrust better.

Standing. This is easiest to perform when both partners are of a similar height. The man can approach from either the rear or the front. If rear entry is desired, it helps for the woman to lean on a table or counter. If front entry is chosen, then it helps for the woman or man to lean against a wall or tree or other object that will help support their weight. Sex while standing can be very spontaneous (we see it all the time in the movies—the love scenes where the couple can't wait, so he hikes up her dress and they go at it behind the office building or in the park against one of the trees). The standing position is fun, but it requires a lot of work and is more appropriate when you just want to have fun rather than work with sex magic.

Seated. We see this position in many statues of Shakti and Shiva. The most usual variation is for the man to sit in a cross-legged position, with the woman sitting in his lap, her legs wrapped around his waist. Other variations have the man sitting on a chair while the woman sits on his lap, facing away from him as she slides down on his penis. These positions can be fun, but they limit the man's movement more than other positions. They are also best when the woman is lighter weight than the man.

Within these basic positions, there are hundreds of variations. If you are a connoisseur and would love to try them all out, I recommend that you buy a copy of the *Kama Sutra* or another sexual positions manual. The most important thing is for both partners to be comfortable in, and aroused by, the sexual position.

Before the Afterglow

One thing I learned about myself that I think may be true for many women is that I can have my most intense orgasms after intercourse. This usually happens when we aren't practicing sacred sex but are "just" going at it—having fun having sex, and not worrying about reaching any goal except our mutual enjoyment.

It's almost as if the foreplay and the fucking build up to a point where I release but don't quite let go of the sexual tension. I am multiorgasmic, so I can come and then build up again once, twice, or more depending on how long we are in the bedroom (or wherever we choose to be at that time).

If I still feel a little pent up afterward, we'll cuddle for a bit, then Sam will use a vibrator on me, and within five minutes, I'll have an explosive orgasm that totally relaxes me. You might want to explore this with your partner. It can make for one more way to increase enjoyment—the woman can have a powerful and grounding orgasm; the man can see just how much added pleasure he can give to his partner.

Afterglow

Afterglow is the common term given to that period of time right after sexual intercourse when the partners haven't quite reentered the world around them, but are still basking in their contentment together. Sometimes reality forces a different schedule on you, but when you can, take the time after sex to linger together in the nude, comfy and safe.

Don't analyze what happened between you at this point. Keep those discussions out of the bedroom, though it may be comforting to your partner to reinforce how much you enjoyed yourself. Just touch softly, chat about unimportant stuff, things that are silly, fun, happy, relaxing.

This is a good time to let the cats (or dogs) onto the bed for family time. We lock our cats out of the bedroom when we're having sex because they get too inquisitive, and there's nothing more distracting than looking over and seeing a fuzzy face with big round eyes staring at you. Afterward, we open the door, and the cats come in and lounge on the bed with us.

The afterglow period can be especially strong when you're practicing sexual communion, and it helps to ground you as you slowly return to this world, so try not to skip it. Make it part of your practice. If sex is worth spending time on, then reinforcing that sense of commitment and contentment and magic is also worth spending time on.

Magic and Sex

As with masturbation, there are ways you can use the energy of orgasm in your magic with your partner. Much of the following reiterates what I wrote in chapter 3, but I've adjusted the process for a couple.

First, you must have a focus for your magic. When you are casting a spell as a couple, it's best to have a common focus that benefits you both or that benefits the earth. If you use your orgasmic energy for someone else, you run the risk of keying into their lives, which could cause havoc in your relationship. Perhaps you both want to focus on one of you getting a coveted job, or on finding that family home you've been looking to buy. Or maybe the local wildlife center needs some financial help, and you'd like to send some powerful energy toward that.

Candle magic is extremely effective for sex magic, but feel free to experiment. Choose two candles, one to represent each of you, preferably an image candle or yoni and lingam candles, but tapers or votives will work also. Follow the instructions for masturbation candle magic. Anoint the candles with your vaginal juices and semen. Let them dry, carve them with appropriate runes, anoint them with a drop or two of your blood or oils to match the energy of your spell, roll them in spell powder if you like, and fasten them into a candle holder. Set up an altar, then cast a Circle and invoke the elements.

Invoke whichever deities you have decided to work with, if you want to work with any. It helps, when you are working as a couple, to invoke a paired set of gods so their energy meshes. Be sure and research your choice thoroughly, especially when working with sex magic. Play music to fit your mood; dance for one another if you like—stripping or erotic dance is a wonderful gift to give your partner.

Turn on the music, light your candles, and spend a little time sliding into the mindset for what you are doing. When you begin to arouse one another, try to keep the focus of your spell in your minds. Use the plateau method we discussed earlier to build up your energy. See it rise just as it does when you create a cone of power. When you are at the point where you can't stop yourselves—when you are going to climax—send the energy rushing toward your magical objective.

With couples work, you should try to time your orgasms together, which is another reason for using the plateau method. This will allow you to catch up to each other.

Afterward, rest in the energy a while before you devoke the elements and deities. Let your candles burn all the way out, and then dispose of the wax remnants.

The magical energy we use in spellcasting is directly connected to the energy of the Kundalini. We can make use of that connection in our magic and in our passionate selves.

Making Time for Sex—Magical or Not

Whether you are just horny and hot or you are about to have the most intense connection with the gods that you've ever had, making time for your sex life is a vital part of any relationship. I maintain that a platonic marriage or love affair can only go so far in uniting a couple. Adaptations may be needed if one or both members are disabled or distance is a factor.

But it comes down to this: When you commit to a physical relationship such as marriage (with or without the benefit of legalities or handfasting), you are committing to more than a friendship. You have a responsibility to help your partner explore and enhance their relationship with their body and with yours. And they have that same responsibility to you.

"How can we schedule more time for sex in our busy lives?" you may ask. Or another common concern is, "What do we do with the kids while we're supposed to be getting down with each other?"

There are several ways you can approach it. If you have to, write an appointment into your calendar. It isn't romantic, but if you treat it as a serious commitment, like any other meeting, then you will be respecting its importance in your lives. You might choose to set aside one night per week to spend as a couple and lock the doors and tell your friends not to come over. You don't always have to have sex on this night. You can watch a movie or go out to dinner, but make sure you are doing something together as a couple.

If you have children and you can't afford a baby-sitter, see if you can trade duties once a week with another couple who has a child and is on a tight budget, so you can both have an evening free every week. If the kids are old enough, drive them to a double feature and spend that time together until you have to pick them up. Or, if you have talked to your children about sex, tell them, "Mom and Dad need some private time. If it's an emergency, you may interrupt us (and list out what the emergencies can be).

Otherwise, you are expected to watch television, read a book, or go play in your room."

Think of other ways to carve out private time together. Do you really need to go to that party Friday night? Does the house have to be spotless, or can you let the vacuuming go for an evening? Four-course gourmet meals are fun to prepare, but maybe you can ease up on their frequency and devote that time to your sex life. Too tired before you turn in for the night? Get up an hour early and enjoy some morning sex. Or put a frozen casserole in the oven, and grab some time for sex while you are waiting for dinner. Meet somewhere for lunch, but have the main course in a hotel room or a locked office and grab a sandwich on the way back to work.

When you are practicing sexual communion exercises, you will need more time; plan on an hour and a half or more. But you don't need to do this every time you have sex. You can revel in the pure joy of lust for its own sake. Perhaps make an agreement to practice sex magic twice a month, maybe on the full and new moons, and devote other times to play.

Uniting the Jade Scepter and the Sacred Lotus

He approaches her naked body, his lingam erect, thrusting upward, the jade scepter of the gods. She dances before him, breasts heavy and ripe, hips curving, swaying to the music that haunts their ears. A rushing in his ears clouds his thoughts; he cannot think. He desires only this most beautiful woman who entices him forward.

She thrusts her hips in circles, coiling like a snake to the music as her hair flies in the candlelit room. The throbbing drumbeat has captured her heart, she must match her body to the beat. She sees him watching her, creeping around the edges of the candle flame's glow, and her pulse quickens. He is the hunter; she is the quarry. But as she twists in rhythm to the driving cadence, she becomes the

162

hunter, the spider weaving the web, and he the quarry. Trading places, trading roles, they encircle one another, eyes ever locked, bodies in constant motion.

In and out, they weave their dance, his cock firm and hard, her pussy wet and aching. And then they are wheeling through the universe, with Shiva, the Blue God, dancing behind them. Shakti's fire races through their feet, hips, arms, hearts, sparking the rhythm and lighting up the sky. They come together, joining, and his jade scepter slides deep within her sacred lotus, and the cycle of the universe is perpetuated.

The union of male and female mirrors the oldest energy of all, that of the primal opposites coming out of the genderless, passive energy that permeates the universe from which we draw all connections and life. Fire and water, yang and yin, we see this pairing in both battle and lovemaking, as the active sparks the passive and a new creation is born.

Though you don't need both male and female to practice sexual communion, the divine marriage, the mating dance of the God and Goddess, has a unified, balanced energy with a man and a woman.

The exercises in this chapter are a process that is more important, in some aspects, than the result. Divine communion is a pathway, not an end unto itself. Through the journey, we learn about ourselves and our partners. As you become more adept, you will create your own rituals that will lead you into a deeper bond not only with each other, but with the very foundations of the divine feminine and masculine. This goes beyond a structured ritual, into the depths of ecstasy and experience, for which there are no guide maps.

I offer you a challenge, as a couple. Spend the next few months focusing on your sex life. Practice the sexual communion exercises and the other exercises in the book. See where the journey takes you. If you make this study, this quest, a priority, you will emerge changed and with a deeper understanding of yourself and your relationships. Through our own research and experiments, Samwise and I have strengthened our marriage, and our sex life, which was good, has become wonderful. We are closer and happier together than we've ever been.

CHAPTER EIGHT

Sex and Magic:
The Divine Marriage

Feel the pulse of the earth,
hear the beat of the cosmos.

DHYANI YWAHOO

The Hieros Gamos is another name for the divine marriage, or sacred marriage. In many magical traditions, this is practiced as an actual or symbolic rite, especially on Sabbats (holidays) like Beltane. Sex creates a psychic bond. Any sexual act performed in a Circle, as representatives of the Gods, will create a bond tighter than any fling or affair with your next-door neighbor. Before you run off and attempt to reenact the Great Rite with a person you just met during a public ritual, think twice.

The Symbolic Hieros Gamos

I'm going to present two rituals for divine marriage. One is the symbolic Hieros Gamos, and the second is an actual Great Rite. Personally, I find the concept of a formal Great Rite too detached and theatrical after all the sex magic I've done with Samwise. However, if I ignore them in this book, I know I'm going to get letters asking why I left the information out.

I urge you, if you are participating in either rite (especially the actual Great Rite), please know your partner and be certain that you can handle the connection this type of ritual can create.

For the symbolic Hieros Gamos, which usually takes place during a larger ceremony (most often the Beltane Sabbat), you will need a chalice of wine and an athame. The Priest holds the athame; the Priestess holds the chalice. Once the Circle has been cast, the elements have been invoked, and the group ritual has taken place, you may begin.

Priestess: (lifts the chalice skyward) I bless this chalice of wine in the name of the Goddess, that it might represent the divine womb of the world and the womb of every female who walks upon this planet, be she animal, bird, reptile, or mortal. Let this chalice of wine represent the nature of the feminine.

Priest: (lifts the athame skyward) I bless this athame in the name of the Horned God, that it might represent the divine phallus of the world and the phallus of every male who walks upon this planet, be he animal, bird, reptile, or mortal. Let this athame represent the nature of the masculine.

Priestess: (bows to the Priest) Without the masculine, there would be no seed to spark life. I honor the God within you.

Priest: (bows to the Priestess) Without the feminine, there would be no egg to receive the seed and no womb to nurture the egg into life. I honor the Goddess within you.

Priestess: (holds out the chalice toward the Priest) The Lady desires the Lord; her yoni opens moist with her passion.

166

Priest: (holds the athame, point down, above the chalice) The Lord desires the Lady; his lingam rises erect with his passion.

Priestess: As the chalice is to the Goddess . . .

Priest: (slowly lowers the athame into the wine) So the athame is to the God. The Lord enters the Lady and joins with her in the sacred marriage.

Priestess: The dance of life begins once more, and so the world shakes with their love and their passion.

Priest: (slowly lifts the athame out of the wine and places it on the altar) And so it is done.

Priestess: Drink now of the sacred union (lifts the chalace to the Priest's lips and helps him sip) You are blessed in the sight of the Gods.

Priest: (takes the chalice and lifts it to the Priestess's lips and helps her sip) Drink now of the sacred union. You are blessed in the sight of the Gods.

Priestess and Priest: (Take the chalice and make the rounds of the Circle, if they are working in a Circle, so everyone can sip from the chalice while the Priest and Priestess bless them in the name of the Gods.)

This ceremony can be done by a solitary practitioner, by adapting both parts, to celebrate Beltane or some other significant holiday. It can also be performed as is or with alterations for your group in a coven setting.

Having personally felt the connection the symbolic Hieros Gamos can create, I recommend that the Priest and Priestess have a close relationship.

The Great Rite

Like the symbolic Hieros Gamos, the actual Great Rite is usually part of a larger ceremony. Sometimes it is used for a magical purpose, such as spellwork. Most often, it's used as part of a ceremony, usually a Sabbat like Beltane. Once again, I caution about the connections that sexual energy can form during magic and ritual. Please stop and think before agreeing to join any ritual about which you are uncertain, or where you don't fully understand what's expected of you. This is true for any magical practice, sexual or not. Such a decision can have serious repercussions.

There can be many variations of this rite. I present the way I would choose to perform the Great Rite, if I were so inclined to focus my sex magic in this direction.

If you are in a group where some members are new or some might be uncomfortable watching another couple have sex, I recommend that you partition an area for the couple who will be enacting the Rite. Once again, I highly recommend that the couple assuming the roles of Priest and Priestess for this Rite be lovers in the "everyday" world, too. If they are not, I suggest that they be single or in polyamorous relationships.

Both members of the couple chosen to perform this rite should feel comfortable with their bodies, and there must be some spark of attraction between them. You don't want to be in the middle of a Great Rite with a dozen people watching and not be able to get it up. If you are the Priestess, you certainly need to feel comfortable with the Priest touching you. The rest of the group must also be comfortable enough with nudity and various body types not to snicker or titter or emanate negative energy toward the couple. If any of these issues concern you, you should make sure the couple has privacy for the Rite.

The group should decide, *before the ritual*, what they will be doing during the Priest and Priestess's sexual union. Will you chant? Visualize? Meditate? How will the group handle their arousal at the sight of a couple having sex? When you're working skyclad, this arousal can be embarrassing. While most groups I've encountered don't operate this way, you must decide whether you want others to participate in sexual activity while the Priest and Priestess are performing the Rite. These are some of the many variables you must work out in advance, or you could end up with a very odd and awkward situation, which, if bad enough, could destroy the group's trust.

You must also address practical matters such as birth control and STDs. Magical energy is the energy of creation, and if you rely on luck to avoid a pregnancy, chances are you're going to come up snake eyes. STDs, as we discussed earlier, are common and can be deadly. Don't ever trust anyone blindly; that could jeopardize your life or your health or your regular partner's life. Work a condom into the ritual!

If the Great Rite is hidden behind a screen or curtains, it may be easier to focus the group's energy. Group members should center their attention on the couple, feeding them with the magic that they are building through the ritual. The couple will channel that energy into their lovemaking and offer it up to the Gods or aim it toward the intent of the spell being cast.

Once the Circle has been cast, the elements have been invoked, and the larger ritual is underway, you may begin. The group (or couple, if this is a private ritual between two people only) is skyclad. A cushioned bed area in the center of the Circle is draped with pillows and scarves that are soft and smooth, not scratchy. The Priestess steps to the center of the group, next to the bed, and stretches her arms to the sides, up above her head (commonly known as the drawing down position). The Priest steps up to her.

Priest: I bow to thee (name of Priestess), you who stand here today, representing the Goddess incarnate. You, who in your power and wisdom, mirror the power and wisdom of the Goddess divine. Will you have me for your partner, to reenact that greatest rite of all between woman and man, to reenact the dance of Shakti and Shiva as they create the universe anew?

Priestess: I will have you (name of Priest), you who stand here today, representing the God incarnate. You, who in your strength and sagacity, mirror the strength and sagacity of the God divine. I will reenact with you that greatest rite of all between man and woman, the dance of Shiva and Shakti as they create the universe anew.

Priest: The fivefold kiss, I bring to thee.

(kisses her lips) I kiss your lips, from which words of wisdom flow.

(kisses her breasts) I kiss your breasts, which feed the world in its birth.

(kisses her groin) I kiss your womb, from which all life emerges.

(kisses her knees) I kiss your knees, which bend before the might of the Universe.

(kisses her feet) I kiss your feet, which walk the paths of the natural order.

(stands again) Priestess (name), you are the altar of the Goddess, your body the temple of the Divine. May I enter your sacred gardens?

Priestess: (lays on the bed) Enter and be welcome, my Lord.

Priest and Priestess: (Proceed to the sexual act, including foreplay. Remember, sex isn't just intercourse.)

The rest of the coven should proceed with their agreed-upon part of the ceremony. When the Priest and Priestess climax and are finished, they will return to the group, and the ritual will proceed as planned. Cakes and wine will be passed and the Circle devoked.

Plowing the Furrow: A Freeform Fertility Ritual

During spring, we honor the returning life to the earth. What better way to revere the Gods and the burgeoning life that is beginning to show through the chill and mist than to do as our ancestors did. This can be done in a group rite, if everyone in the group is comfortable with the idea, or by a solitary couple.

Find a spot out in nature. Whether or not it is a plowed field isn't important. Look for privacy, safety, and a lack of poisonous plants and bugs. This would be an excellent ritual for blessing a garden before you plant seeds. Just make sure that your neighbors aren't getting an eyeful.

Bring a tape recorder, some magical, sensuous instrumental music, wine or nonalcoholic grape juice to toast the Gods, cakes for the Gods, food to share after the rite, condoms, towels, and washcloths. Wear clothes that can get dirty. Cast a Circle and invoke the elements. Invoke whichever deities you choose to work with; however in this ritual, deities connected with the earth or creation would be your best choices.

Priestess: In days of old, we came together to bless the earth with fertility in the name of the Gods. We joined in the dance of life, in the passion of the divine union that our energy might help the turning of the Wheel and the growth of new life.

Priest: So is it now, that we come together in the fields to show our love and reverence for this most ancient of traditions. The plow of the God delves deep into the womb of the Goddess, planting seed that the cycle might turn once again.

Priestess: (holds up the bottle of wine) Blessings to the Lady and Lord, from their sacred vineyard. (pours wine onto the earth)

Priest: (holds up ritual cakes) Blessings to the Lady and Lord, from their sacred fields. (crumbles cakes onto the earth)

Priestess: Dance! Dance all; join in ecstasy and passion. Give back to the earth even as the earth gives to you.

Turn on the music. Everyone should start dancing skyclad as partners gradually move together. Empowered by the rut of the stag, the man should seek his mate. Empowered by the drive of the Sacred Harlot, the woman should seek her mate. Partners come together in passion on the ground, naked in the soft folds of the earth, and channeling energy into the soil, giving their orgasm and passion to the Lord and Lady.

After the ritual, light a bonfire, if you can, and toast bread and meat for your dinner. Eat fruit and sweets, drink, and rejoice in the ecstasy of the body as well as the ecstasy of the soul.

CHAPTER NINE

Straight As a Slinky: Kink, Gender Preference, Polyamory, and Pagans

> Yasmine: "You're straight as a Slinky, doll."
> Bob: "So are you. You just won't admit it yet."
>
> CONVERSATION, 1989

When I was eight years old, my Barbie dolls tied each other up, flogged each other, and had lesbian sex. I didn't own any Ken dolls. He didn't have genitals, and I knew *that* was wrong. When I was thirteen, I began a play called *Dear Uncle William* (of course it would star Roddy McDowell, who I had a crush on at that time) about a newlywed couple who went to visit the groom's odd uncle in an old castle in England. Dear Uncle William killed his nephew, chained the bride to the bed, whipped her, and had sex with her. She liked it even though she hated him. After about twenty pages, I got bored so I quit writing that particular play and started a new one that was a thinly veiled remake of *Planet of the Apes*.

In my first year at Evergreen State College, shortly after I entered the Craft, a woman made a pass at me and I freaked. I'm sure it's because I sensed, somewhere deep inside, that I *was* interested. By this time my sex-

173

ual fantasies seemed firmly entrenched in the bizarre, and I couldn't talk to anyone about them. The last thing I needed was to feel that I was any farther out on the fringe. Thinking that I might have lesbian or bisexual tendencies was more than I could handle at the time.

During my twenties, however, I was in a bad relationship, and the sex was almost nonexistent. I fantasized a lot at this time, and I had to admit to myself that at least 50 percent of my fantasies were about women. The other half, the fantasies with men in them, were far from idyllic romantic escapades. While I was not familiar with the term at that time, they were firmly in the BDSM realm.

I was working for the state in 1989, when I met a man whom I'll call Bob. From the first day I started work in his department, we connected. We had barely spoken when he asked, "So, do you work in white, gray, or black?" I realized my pentacle was hanging down inside my dress and he couldn't see it, but he still knew that I was a Witch. As I smiled and said, "Gray," I knew this was going to be an interesting friendship.

He wasn't my type, yet he appealed to me. He flirted with me all the time and seemed to know every trigger to every button I had. Though he was never offensive, it was clear that he was trying to entice me into an affair. I was desperately clinging to the last vestiges of my marriage and kept dodging his attention.

One day Bob walked up behind me and whispered, "I can make you melt."

Angry at myself because I found it difficult to ignore my reactions to his energy, I said, "I don't think so. I'm the queen of ice."

He came back with, "That's easy to take care of. All I have to do is raise the temperature a little bit, and ice melts."

A few days later he invited me to his apartment for lunch and, against my better judgment, I went with him. We really did enjoy each other's company, and he was a breath of fresh air in a stale work environment. When we were at his apartment, we ate lunch and then sat down to talk. He told me that he'd just bought a new paddle for his toybox; would I like to see it? I stared at him, speechless, as he went on to suggest that we call in sick for the afternoon and spend the time playing.

Let me tell you, that was the hardest refusal I've ever had to make. I wanted to stay. I wanted to fuck him. I wanted to explore this toybox of his (having never met anyone else who admitted having one). I wanted to taste the world that I sensed he lived in. But my loyalty to my marriage won out, and I thanked him for the offer but declined. He was disappointed, but soon after he found a boyfriend, and I learned that he was bisexual. With his attentions occupied elsewhere, I found myself more than a little jealous, though I had no right to be.

A year or so later, I was out of my relationship and edging ever closer to the truth about myself. I met a woman with whom I became close friends. She moved in as my roommate. We never seemed to get her bed set up, so she just slept in mine. During a wild summer of magic, we became lovers. Within the space of one night, my view of myself shifted. I finally accepted that I was bisexual. When I met Sam, my bisexuality didn't play into my decision to marry him. I simply fell in love with the person, not the gender.

Accepting my need for BDSM took me a few more years. When a friend got into it and came out openly about her interest, my reaction was so strong that I realized my feelings were probably coming from fear about facing my own desires. A year or so later, I finally faced the full truth of my nature.

I have come to a place where I revel in the fact that I, too, am "straight as a Slinky." I never dreamed that I'd someday describe myself that way. But Bob knew. I suppose like recognizes like.

In this chapter, we look at alternative perceptions of sexuality, namely kink (BDSM). While not all who involve themselves in these activities are Pagan, the activities lend themselves easily to the Pagan lifestyle.

Pagans differ from the majority of society by honoring sex as a wonderful, natural part of life and accepting a diversity of sexual play and sexual preference. Our belief structure is, for the most part, founded on the sexual union of the God and Goddess. Through the cycles and the Wheel of the Year, the seasons flow, growth leads into harvest into fallow periods, and birth leads to death to birth again. Sex, in all its forms, is a sacred and ritual act, and it is also play and fun and a good fuck. If there is one credo we tend to agree on it's: safe, sane, and consensual.

BDSM

Tonight, as we are sitting on the bed, kissing, I can feel a familiar need rise up in me. I've been in my head too much lately and can't quit thinking, can't quite focus on the feel of his lips on my skin. I've been too busy lately, too caught up in my work and the various responsibilities that are my dubious honor to carry out.

"Would you tie me up?" I quietly ask. Samwise smiles; he understands what I am asking. It took us many talks to help him see what I wanted, but finally he understood my view and became comfortable with his role during the times I need this.

He takes the velvet rope from the hook above our bed and lovingly binds my wrists, then hangs the rope over the hook so my arms are above my head.

The soft kiss of the velvet combined with the strength of the knots is exquisitely erotic, and the moment the material touches my skin, I feel a drop in my stomach; my arousal flares. When my hands are bound, I lose my need to control. Though I know he would stop if I asked him to, this allows me to release my ever-active mind. I am free from the drive to decide, to be the aggressor in life that I am.

With my hands tied, every touch on my flesh is heightened. His attention centers on my pleasure; bound, I cannot return the favor. I am passive, receptive, totally yin. He runs a flail lightly over my body. It tickles, and I laugh in joyous freedom. The licks from the leather strips are stimulating. I let my mind roam free, and I head for the place of the flowers.

BDSM is a catchall phrase for a number of sexual (and sometimes nonsexual) activities. Its adherents simply call it "kink." Numerous misconceptions surround these activities. Many people are actively involved in aspects of BDSM, and the more we bring it out of the closet, the more we can separate the ideas of consensual play from abuse. While a lot of BDSMer's enjoy vanilla sex on occasion (the term for nonkinky and non-spiritually oriented sex), most prefer to mingle kink with the majority of their erotic activities.

BDSM stands for bondage, domination, and sadomasochism. These practices are generally grouped as bondage and discipline, domination and submission, and sadomasochism.

B&D—bondage and discipline (sometimes called bondage and domination). This practice focuses on physical restraint. I think one of the best descriptions I've read for the psychology behind this (and it includes my own attraction to being bound) was in an interview in *Different Loving*, the book that has practically become the bible for BDSM. Cléo Dubois is a rather well-known dominatrix and the partner of Fakir Musafar, who is considered one of the founders of the Modern Primitive Movement. Dubois says, "A lot of people want bondage. I had a friend who said that when the ropes are on the outside, the ropes on the inside get loose. When you're tied up, you can be free. I really understand that dynamic. If you're tied up, you're no longer responsible. Bondage gives you permission to let go. It's a paradox: If you are helpless, you are actually freer."

Restraints seldom include the handcuff props that are often promoted for bondage play by those who do not understand these activities. There are many types of bondage, some of which have become art forms.

Bonds include everything from silk scarves to leather wrist cuffs to rope. Mummification may use Saran wrap, sheets, ace bandages, or other wrapping materials. Mummification is an extreme form of sensory deprivation that should not be attempted without a knowledgeable guide and mentor. Oriental bondage uses rope, and the knots are intricate, uniform, and generally symmetrical. There are specific restraints for various body parts too, such as for breast bondage or cock-and-ball bondage.

Another form of restraint is the blindfold. This forces the attention inward, on the body, so helps you remove yourself from the outer world and all the cares, worries, and tasks that await you.

D&S—domination and submission. This practice has one partner act dominant and the other act submissive during erotic play or as a lifestyle choice. Strong-natured people need a place to give up their sense of responsibility, and some do so in the bedroom, letting their vulnerability reign.

People who are lifestyle D&Ser's carry this master/slave or top/sub relationship into their daily life. Their natures conform happily to these roles. Bondage can be used, at times, in this type of relationship, though D&S tends to focus on a control of the mind rather than the body. Discipline is also practiced, both mental and physical. Misbehavior will be punished.

S&M—sadomasochism. Pain and punishment can be used in a consensual manner for erotic purposes. True S&M is not forced onto unwilling partners. In *Screw the Roses, Send Me the Thorns*, Phillip Miller and Molly Devon say, "*SM IS NOT ABUSE!* Things that make our partners unhappy are bad things and we leave them alone. We don't do things to our partners without their permission or because we are mad at each other. Abusive people do not ask for permission and act out of anger, and they sure as hell don't negotiate a beating. The things we do to each other are done solely in the divine spirit of love and lust."

Sadomasochism is another method for transcending the limitations we set for ourselves, for training the body to carry the mind to ecstatic highs. Ritual pain was common in many aboriginal rites. I know several people who use S&M in this manner. The punishments, or disciplines, in S&M range from spanking to flogging to more intense activities. Nothing is done, however, that isn't agreed on beforehand. Someone truly versed in S&M will never force you into a situation to which you object.

Other Kinky Activities

The kink scene includes a number of other sexual and erotic activities. Some may find a spiritual use for these, others will not. Since I do not have a firm grounding in most of these, I simply present a few for you to research further if you're interested.

Anal sex. Common among gay men, this is also practiced by some heterosexual and lesbian couples. Proponents say that anal sex is better for the man because the anal passage is tighter than the vagina and therefore feels better. They also claim that if performed correctly, it should not be painful. One must go slowly, however. Rushing during anal sex is likely to tear the delicate muscles, and infection is much more common with this practice than it is in "regular" sex.

Feminization. This is the practice of feminizing men who are active submissives. This can include dressing them in women's clothing, taping their genitals tightly, or forcing them to assume a feminine role in the relationship.

Pony training. In this practice, a submissive is taught to assume the role of a well-trained horse (as in Anne Rice's *Sleeping Beauty* series) for their master or mistress. Some pony boys and girls are actively ridden, and their "owners" may buy a saddle for the pony. Others may be trained to pull carts (usually they are standing while wearing a harness attached to the cart) and to step proudly—like a show horse.

Corseting. A corset restricts the waist, which helps to modify and control the body. This is actually a form of body modification, though many connect it to sexuality.

If You Wish to Pursue BDSM

If you find that BDSM resonates with you and you wish to pursue it as an active part of your life, or even as an avenue of study, here are some basic suggestions to guide you through the labyrinth of this subculture.

- Remember the basic rule that all BDSMer's embrace: Safe, Sane, and Consensual. In other words, you had better not do anything to your partner that they don't agree with. On the flip side, if your partner overstep your boundaries, stop them immediately.

- Create a safe word. When you say this word, your partner knows that they are going too far, hurting you in a way not agreed upon, or that something else is wrong. This word shouldn't be a common word, especially not the word "no" because that's used so often during sexual excitement that you'd have your partner stopping every five minutes in an intense scene. On the other hand, it must be a word that is easy to remember. It's doubtful that you could wrap your mind around "proletariat" when someone's spanking you too hard.

- Know your play partner. If you meet someone who claims to be an expert master, who promises you delights beyond your imagination, how do you know that he or she isn't psychotic or inexperienced and, therefore, dangerous? Or just full of hot air? Get to know people before you put your trust in them. Study

BDSM, especially if you are interested in the more hardcore activities, such as rope bondage, mummification, or S&M punishments. Read books on the subject, visit websites, and go to bars and fetish gatherings. This will give you an idea of what's out there. In other words: don't be stupid.

What to Do If You Want BDSM and Your Partner Doesn't

This subject is familiar to me. As I said before, Samwise and I went through this scenario. We were lucky in that we were willing to discuss it until we found what works for us as a couple. We're equal partners.

When your partner wants some aspect of BDSM and you are reluctant, or vice versa, there are very few options. Discuss it and see if you can find an acceptable compromise. Be aware, this sort of discussion can take months to iron out. Ultimately, no one should be coerced into something they aren't comfortable with, that they have thought over and know they just can't participate in. Sometimes, through open and honest communication, you will be able to find a middle ground.

But what happens if you can't find a compromise that works for both of you? Can you give up the desire and live without it? For some this will work, for others it won't. You or your partner might decide that this is so important you must pursue the activity outside your relationship. If this happens, you need to discuss where this will leave your relationship. You can either open your marriage or partnership, which is not easy, or you can separate. I never recommend sneaking around behind your partner's back. This is wrong. No ifs, ands, or buts, you owe it to your partner and to yourself to be honest about what you are doing sexually.

These latter choices are major shifts for a relationship and should not be made in haste. If Sam and I had not been able to find a compromise, I'm not sure what we would have done, but I think our love and commitment would have pulled us through. Our sacred sex practices often replace bondage for me, but there are times when that's just not enough. And for those times, I'm not sure how I'd deal with the frustration if that velvet cord wasn't hanging above our bed.

Gender Preference

In our society, homosexuality of any kind is considered suspect, though that viewpoint is easing up a bit. The fight for gay rights continues even as churches condemn the lifestyle and hate crimes rise.

As elsewhere, the Pagan community has had to overcome certain assumptions and expectations of gay and lesbian relationships. In the past, one partner was expected to be very masculine and the other, very feminine. We seem to have moved beyond those stereotypes. There are still flaming gays and bull dykes and their opposites, but not every lesbian or queer fits into a category easily. Above all, we are human and—like all humans—we have myriad aspects of our personalities.

For me, the concept of being bisexual is thus: I love people on an individual basis, regardless of gender, color, or age (within lawful limits). When I was thirty, I was going out with a nineteen-year-old girl. I let her make the first move, and I waited till I was sure she was seriously interested. When I was seventeen, I was involved with a twenty-four-year-old man from India. Attraction will break through where it will, age, color, and sex be damned.

Some people are exclusively oriented toward one sex or another, but I think, when you dig really deep, each person has considered what it would be like to fuck someone of their own gender (or the opposite gender, if you happen to be solidly gay).

I also believe that you can't force yourself to be attracted to someone. You can't turn someone gay just like you can't turn someone another color. Though I've met some pretty obnoxious people, both gay and straight, who thought they could.

"Give me five minutes with that man, and he'd be mine!" A guy I met at a pagan festival actually said this about Samwise. Besides ignoring the fact that Sam is straight and not interested in men, Brownie insulted my ability to keep Samwise happy in bed (by insinuating he could 'turn' Sam gay) he knew Sam was my husband. When he noticed that I'd overheard him, the guy added, "But I wouldn't try it because you'd kick my butt, wouldn't you, sweetie?" I just smiled and said, "Count on it, babe, and believe me, you wouldn't sit down for a month."

On the other side of the coin, I've heard men declare, "Ah, she just hasn't found the right man yet or she'd drop all that gay nonsense. Give me a chance, and I'll set her straight." When my girlfriend and I held hands at a crafts fair one day, we overheard two guys as they walked by. One of them said, "What a waste, goddamn dykes." Not only crude, they were totally ignorant of the basic nature of gender preference.

My tendencies towards bisexuality were strong enough that when my lover approached me, it was the most natural thing in the world for me to respond. If I didn't have those tendencies, or at least the curiosity, I probably wouldn't have consented.

Acceptance Exercise

This exercise is for anyone who is uncomfortable with the idea of touching someone of their own sex. It will not turn you gay; that's a ridiculous premise. It will help you understand the beauty in your own sex and how you might find someone of your own gender sexually attractive.

Collect pictures of people who are your own gender: men if you are male, women if you are female. You will probably need to buy some new magazines or books! They should be nude, in all different colors, shapes, and sizes. Also collect a few pictures of men making love to men or women making love to women.

Set up aside some time in a quiet place where you won't be disturbed. Start by looking at the singular nudes, one by one. Examine them from an artistic point of view. What is beautiful about each body? Bodies have interesting curves and lines. What other shapes do they suggest to you?

Now look at the pictures of couples. How do they make you feel? Are you nervous when you look at these pictures? Do they excite you in any manner; If so, how does this make you feel? Examine your preconceptions about what gay or lesbian sex is like compared to what you see in the pictures.

Return your attention to the pictures of singles. Can you imagine engaging one of these people in a sexual manner? What do you think it would feel like to run your hands over their bodies? Allow your imagination free rein. You may not find this arousing at all, and that's absolutely okay. Perhaps you'll be surprised by your reaction. Try to set aside your prejudgments and assumptions about your own sexuality for this exercise.

Now consider your reactions. If you aren't sexually attracted to your own gender, imagine what it's like for someone who is gay who feels no attraction to the opposite sex. Most television programs, movies, and so on are geared toward opposite-sex attraction. How would you feel if the opposite were true? What if our society focused on same-sex connections? If you are heterosexual, chances are you would feel excluded, as if there was something wrong with your sexual preference. Examine your attitudes and actions for prejudices and discriminatory beliefs.

Though I usually espouse tolerance of other viewpoints, I believe that hate crimes are truly sins. Acts of rape, murder, and torture are often committed simply because of a person's gender, race, or religious or sexual preference. We can't always be politically correct, but we can urge our representatives to create equal opportunities and conditions for all. We can actively work toward a society where anyone can get married, regardless of gender preference, where we can denounce hate crimes for the bigoted and perverse acts that they are.

Gender Preference and the Divine

Within the Pagan community, bisexuality and homosexuality are generally accepted. However, for a long time that wasn't true, particularly among some of the more traditional forms of Wicca and Witchcraft. The polarity of the God and Goddess were seen as the only natural communion. In the last twenty years, this has changed, especially with the rise of Dianic groups and fairy covens—and we ain't talking about the faerie realm here.

Dianic Witchcraft tends to be unipolar, recognizing only the Goddess. Much of this is a reaction to the patriarchal dominance that has ruled us for so long. Some Dianics are militant man haters, not a good thing, while others simply want to practice magic focused on female energy. A few view the world through revisionist history, ignoring fact and replacing it with supposition about the history of our Pagan ancestors, especially women's roles and rights. This is also true of a number of modern Wiccans and Witches, regardless of gender preference.

Gay groups practicing magic do not seem to have as negative a view of the Goddess as Dianics have of the God, though their focus is, of course, on Pan and some of the other bisexual or homosexual deities and practices.

I have found that mixed groups work fine. A combination of straight, bisexual, and gay or lesbian men and women will not create friction when working magic together. It does become noticeable when you work sex magic because the energy is different than a polar male-female blend.

A number of the aboriginal shamans were and are bisexual, and they used practices from shape shifting to bondage and pain to transcend the mundane and reach for the Divine. Bisexuality was inherent to some of the shamanistic systems, perhaps because they were better able to comprehend nature and life when they were intimate with all its people. To understand humans as a whole, you have to understand the opposite gender in addition to your own. Bisexuality can help with this. I am a woman, and by loving women I get a glimpse of why men are attracted to us, though the attraction is not precisely the same.

Alternative sexuality is mirrored in a number of deities. Pombagira, the Brazilian sacred harlot, is the God or Goddess (alternately) of transvestites, homosexuals, and prostitutes. Turquoise Woman, an American Indian Goddess frequently mentioned in Navaho myth, was a bisexual (both sexes) creator/creatrix. And we know Hermaphrodite, the son of Hermes and Aphrodite, who took on the nature of both sexes. There are also a number of deities who took both male and female lovers, Pan and Diana being two of the most celebrated for this.

Humans have both masculine and feminine aspects. We can find the polarity of the God and the Goddess within ourselves. Whether we unite in opposite-sex or same-sex relationships, we can all celebrate and commune with the divine.

Lovers of Artemis Ritual: A Celebration of the Feminine

Since Artemis, Greek Goddess of the Hunt, is often revered in Dianic groups, we are going to invoke her for the central focus of this ritual. This ceremony can be performed by either a solitary lesbian or bisexual practitioner, or by lovers; adapt it as necessary for the number of participants. Try to schedule this ritual for the waxing or full moon. Set up your altar with some or all of the following: fern, ivy, white roses, white carnations, silver and quartz, a statue of Artemis, a crystal bowl with lightly tinted water in it, antlers if you have them, and a bow and arrow. You will need a chalice of wine or grape juice and either dates and fruits and/or cookies and chocolate on the altar. You will also need oil that reflects the aspects of Artemis. Dress in white or earth tones, though your clothes will be coming off so you can begin skyclad if you like.

Cast a Circle, and invoke the elements. Then invoke Artemis:

Lady of the Moon, you who are full and brilliant, you who shine down from your abode in the heavens, hear us! Be with us in our rites, as we celebrate our feminine natures and the very essence of womanhood. The woodland is your home, the moon your bed, and the night and the stars are your colors. We welcome you, great Artemis, with love and blessings.

Take off your clothes. Say, "As we were naked at birth, so we remove our clothing now to stand before the Goddess. With no shame, no guilt, simply joy in our bodies as they are in all their myriad forms of beauty." Everyone should follow suit.

Raise the chalice and say, "Bless this wine, the blood of the Goddess that flows from her womb each month." Draw an invoking pentacle over the chalice, then sip and pass it to each person.

Raise the plate of sweets and say, "Bless these sweetmeats, for they come from the body of the Goddess, upon which we stand and live." Draw an invoking pentacle over the sweets, then take one and pass the plate to each person.

The person acting as Priestess will lead the litany if this is a group. If solitary, then you will be the only priestess. If a couple is performing this ritual, they can take turns.

Hold up the bottle of goddess oil. Say, "Blessed be in the name of Great Artemis, goddess of the Night, the Moon, and the Hunt." Then anoint every woman present between her breasts and begin the litany. If this is a group ritual, this should be a call-and-response rite, with the group repeating each blessing after the Priestess.

Hail and blessed be our feet, that walk the paths of the Goddess.

Hail and blessed be our knees, that kneel at her altar.

Hail and blessed be our clits, which give us much pleasure.

Hail and blessed be our vaginas, the tunnels that usher new life into this world.

187

Hail and blessed be our wombs, that nurture life from a spark, an egg, and seed.

Hail and blessed be our breasts, that suckle and give nourishment.

Hail and blessed be our hearts, that feel the joys and sorrows of mortal life.

Hail and blessed be our hands, with which we create, form and shape our world.

Hail and blessed be our lips, with which we communicate.

Hail and blessed be our eyes, with which we view the world.

Hail and blessed be our minds, with which we think, reason, and imagine.

Hail and blessed be our souls, with which we touch the realms of the Gods.

After the litany, each woman should turn to the woman on her left, in turn, and give her a kiss. This may be passionate or not.

Next, the Priestess should step in the center of the Circle and say, "I celebrate my womanhood and rejoice in my (fill in the blank—this could be something as fundamental as 'good fortune' or as lofty as 'love of life')." When the Priestess steps out of the Circle, the next woman takes her turn.

When all have finished, the Priestess takes her place in the center again and says, "We celebrate the love of woman for woman, of women for the Goddess, of the Goddess for women. We come together to rejoice in our femininity, in our strength as women, in our power and beauty, in our brilliance and wisdom."

If the group is not sexually involved, you can end the ritual here and devoke Artemis and the elements and open the Circle. If the group is sexually intimate, you can go on and turn the energy into passion, making love in the presence of the Goddess. If you are practicing this alone, you might wish to masturbate to orgasm to celebrate the energy of the Goddess and the joy of being in your body as a woman this time.

This ritual reaffirms feminine energy. It is good to practice it on a regular basis alone to remind you of your connection to the divine feminine.

Lovers of Pan Ritual: A Celebration of the Masculine

This ceremony can be performed by either a solitary gay or bisexual practitioner, or by lovers; adapt it as necessary for the number of participants. Try to schedule this ritual for the waxing or full moon. Set up your altar with some or all of the following: fern, ivy, oak leaves, lavender, larkspur, gold and citrine, a statue of Pan, antlers if you have them, and a set of panpipes. You will need a chalice of wine or grape juice and either dates and fruits and/or cookies and chocolate on the altar. You will also need oil that reflects the aspects of Pan. Dress in earth tones, though your clothes will be coming off so you can begin skyclad if you like.

Cast a Circle, and invoke the elements. Then invoke Pan:

> *Lord of the fields, you who are verdant and ripe, you who are the lord of panic and the joy of ecstasy. You who are the haunting call from the woodland and the low trill of fluttering notes from behind the trees, hear us! Be with us in our rites, as we celebrate our masculine natures and the very essence of manhood. The woodland is your home, the moon your light, and the sunlit grove and the trees are your colors. We welcome you, great Pan, with love and blessings.*

Take off your clothes. Say, "As we were naked at birth, so we remove our clothing now to stand before the God. With no shame, no guilt, simply joy in our bodies as they are in all their myriad forms of strength and virility." Everyone should follow suit.

Raise the chalice and say, "Bless this wine, the blood of the God that flows from his veins during harvest." Draw an invoking pentacle over the chalice, then sip and pass it to each person.

Raise the plate of sweets and say, "Bless these sweetmeats, for they come from the body of the God, the spirit of the corn and grain." Draw an invoking pentacle over the sweets, then take one and pass the plate to each person.

The person acting as Priest will lead the litany if this is a group. If solitary, then you will be the only priest. If a couple is performing this ritual, they can take turns.

Hold up the bottle of oil. Say, "Blessed be in the name of Great Pan, lord of the fields, the groves, and music." Then anoint every man present over his heart and begin the litany. If this is a group ritual, this should be a call-and-response rite, with the group repeating each blessing after the Priest.

Hail and blessed be our feet, that walk the paths of the God.

Hail and blessed be our knees, that kneel at his altar.

Hail and blessed be our cocks, which give us much pleasure.

Hail and blessed be our testes, which bring forth the seed of life.

Hail and blessed be our chests, which provide strength for protecting our own.

Hail and blessed be our hearts, that feel the joys and sorrows of mortal life.

Hail and blessed be our hands, with which we create, form, and shape our world.

Hail and blessed be our lips, with which we communicate.

Hail and blessed be our eyes, with which we view the world.

Hail and blessed be our minds, with which we think, reason, and imagine.

Hail and blessed be our souls, with which we touch the realms of the Gods.

After the litany, each man should turn to the man on his left, in turn, and give him a kiss. This may be passionate or not.

Next, the Priest should step in the center of the Circle and say, "I celebrate my manhood and rejoice in my (fill in the blank—this could be something as fundamental as 'good fortune' or as lofty as 'love of life')." When the Priest steps out of the Circle, the next man takes his turn.

When all have finished, the Priest takes his place in the center again and says, "We celebrate the love of man for man, of men for the God, of the God for men. We come together to rejoice in our masculinity, in our strength as men, in our power and beauty, in our brilliance and wisdom."

If the group is not sexually involved, you can end the ritual here and devoke Pan and the elements and open the Circle. If the group is sexually intimate, you can go on and turn the energy into passion, making love in the presence of the God. If you are practicing this alone, you might wish to masturbate to orgasm to celebrate the energy of the God and the joy of being in your body as a man this time.

This ritual reaffirms masculine energy. It is good to practice it on a regular basis alone to remind you of your connection to the divine male.

Group Marriage, Free Love, and One-to-One Commitment

Polyamory is the practice of creating an extended marriage, ranging from triads on up. The Church of All Worlds, an incorporated Pagan church basing its doctrine on Robert Heinlein's *Stranger in a Strange Land*, is a primary proponent of polyamory in the Pagan community, with numerous articles about polyamory on their website.

Obviously, there are enormous hurdles to overcome in this sort of relationship, including jealousy, worry over venereal disease, reaction to public opinion, and trust. You cannot build a successful polyamorous relationship unless your primary relationship is secure. Then you must ask yourself, "Will a third (or fourth) partner want this to be their primary relationship too, and how will we meet those needs if my primary partner doesn't want the relationship to be on an equal basis?" Not all group marriages offer equality within the relationship for all members.

Honesty is vital in a polyamorous relationship. A group marriage has no chance of survival without truthfulness and appropriate damage control when necessary. Honesty is vital for any relationship to be healthy, including your connection to yourself. When you add a third member to a partnership, the potential for trouble increases exponentially. Two people have to cope with two sets of perceptions. When you add a third person, you have created three secondary intimacies within the triad. You have Person A with Person B, A with C, B with C, and the group as a whole. This is an intricate and complex series of connections, and you can imagine the many possibilities for misunderstanding, as well as for pleasure.

I am not a follower of polyamory myself, nor is Samwise. We both feel that a primary relationship is hard enough, and I've seldom known a group marriage scenario that worked for long, though there are a few who say they've found a way to make it last. Most often, a primary couple has a series of short-term partners. Marriage, whether to one person or to many, requires a tremendous amount of work to remain strong and viable.

Some people practice panfidelity. Unlike polyamory, panfidelity does not espouse forming long-term or committed relationships, though practitioners may form a long-term relationship with "no strings attached."

Most polyamorous groups create a system of rules and ethics for themselves. The person who chooses panfidelity usually doesn't want to abide by or create rules, preferring total freedom from the emotional responsibility that accompanies a long-term commitment. Be honest about your desires. Not everyone needs or wants to be in a committed relationship, whether it be a group marriage or a monogamous one. Don't try to force someone into a relationship they do not want.

Monogamy is the most familiar pairing in our society; it's a one-to-one relationship with no outside sexual activity. Strictly insisted on in many religions (including Christianity), monogamy has gotten a bad rap because of the divorce rate and the infidelity rate in our country. However, divorce and infidelity occur for many reasons, and it's too easy to pin these activities on a desire for sexual variety. If you are honest with your partner, if you express your needs and you both work toward a mutually acceptable compromise, monogamy has its own charms. The intimacy of a one-on-one relationship can be incredibly intense.

There are positive and negative points with each type of relationship, and only you can decide what will be right in your life. Whatever you choose, don't mislead others as to where you stand on the issue, and for your own sake, make sure you find out your partner's true feelings before getting deeply involved.

Sexuality is not limited to sweet whisperings in the moonlight and gentle caresses during a night of passion. Neither is it confined to black lace garters and fishnet stockings. Sexuality is as diverse as those who inhabit this planet, as rich as we want it to be, as passionate as our hearts desire. Sexuality is an essential part of our being, and whether we choose to explore it through solitary or interactive means, as human beings, we cannot escape this primal drive.

Enjoy your bodies, find your connection to the Divine through this most ecstatic of gifts. Embrace your passion, and explore the shadows of your sexual being. Self-examination, whether or not we act on what we find, can only lead to greater understanding of ourselves, those around us, and the universe we live in.

CHAPTER TEN

When Sex Is Used As a Weapon: Surviving Rape and Reclaiming Power

A lot of times you shut off your whole heart
from your experience; you close the door,
and you wither and die.

TORI AMOS, INTERVIEW

When I was seventeen and recently graduated from community college, I hitchhiked to California to live with my sister and enjoy life and have adventures. We were finally really getting to know one another. I cherished the moments. I'm glad I did; in less than a decade she'd be dead and I'd have lost her forever.

We went out to bars now and then; they didn't check for my identification. One night we met a couple of guys at a bar, and one of them who went by the name Kitch got the hots for Claudia. He started coming over to visit us. All we knew about him was that he was a Vietnam vet and a cocaine addict.

One evening, we all got drunk. I was lonely; I missed my home state and was tired of living in suburban Los Angeles. Claudia developed a headache, so she went to bed. That left Kitch and me to talk. I couldn't think clearly, but something felt off when he moved closer to me on the sofa. He reached out and grabbed my wrists. I tried to pull away, thinking he was joking, but then he shoved his face close to mine and said, "Want to get raped, honey?"

I really started to fight, but he was a lot stronger than me and I was drunk. The one thought running through my head was that if I screamed, Claudia would come running out and she would kill him; I was sure she'd do it. She'd stab him to death, she'd be sent to jail, her kids wouldn't have a mother, and it would be my fault.

Kitch threw me back against the sofa. I remember my wrists hurting while he held them, as he stuck his tongue down my throat and moved one of his hands down to pull down my panties. The next thing I knew, he was raping me. It only took him a moment to climax, and then he laughed and gave me a kiss on the forehead. I remember he said "Thanks, honey" as he zipped up his pants and grabbed his jacket. "That was fun. We'll have to do it again." He left. I tried to sit up. I wanted to throw up, wanted to crawl into the closet and hide. My sister was still sleeping in the other room. Her kids didn't see; thank gods they were asleep in their room.

I sat on that sofa, crying, still drunk and confused, until I could make myself get up and go take a shower. When I looked in the mirror, my reflection was wrong; I didn't look like me anymore. Something was missing. Kitch didn't beat me, didn't knife me, didn't tear me to bits. He just stole something from me that took me a long time to recover—my dignity and my sense that I belonged to myself.

I've come a long way since that night when I sat there, wondering what I did wrong to end up getting raped. It took me years to tell anyone what had happened to me. I didn't tell my sister until she was dying from cancer, and she asked me why I had never said anything. I told her, quite honestly, that I had believed at the time that I was protecting her and her kids.

Even if I had decided to prosecute, I didn't know his real name. And I was drunk and seventeen. That alone would have tipped the scales in his favor back in 1979. The courts blamed the victims, believing in the evils of women's sexuality.

You wore a short skirt? You asked for it. You slow danced with the guy? It was your fault. You were walking alone at ten in the morning? How can you expect to be safe! Eighty years old and you forgot to lock your apartment door when you went to bed? Well, grandma, see what happens when you're careless? Three years old and he stuck his cock in your mouth? Well, baby, you'll get over it, and anyway, he's just misunderstood; he couldn't help himself because he has a problem so we aren't going to prosecute. You were a bad little boy, and she made you touch her there? Ah come on, be a man; you liked it, you know you did!

Some folks may call me a reactionary; I don't care. The world would be a lot better off without rapists and child molesters. I say we should send them off planet, not as a deterrent, but so the bastards will never be free to do it again. I live in the area that spawned Ted Bundy and the Green River Killer; I know what it's like to be afraid of being alone at night.

But back in 1979 I didn't speak up. I didn't tell anyone. I didn't want to think about it. I just went on with my life, while a small dark blotch covered my heart, a blemish on my soul, and I tried to pretend that it never happened that I was over it. Whenever feelings or thoughts about the rape came up, I repressed them. Two years later I came dangerously close to getting raped again. I went for a walk with a guy I met on campus. He invited me into his apartment to get a drink of water, and when I followed him in, he grabbed me. I got loose, and I stopped going into strange men's apartments. The next year I was hitchhiking and almost didn't escape from a guy who picked me up in a van. Stupid? Yes, and I was still very young. Does that mean I deserved to be raped? No. Absolutely not. I managed to talk my way out of that one, and he let me out on the side of the road. I filed the experience under "R" for "repression."

I knew many women who were raped—date rape and stranger rape and incest and all those horrible assaults. But I wasn't much use to these women as a friend because I was too busy avoiding my own memories.

Years later, in 1992, the Lady decided that it was time I face my fears. I took a self-defense class and discovered that I couldn't scream for help. I physically could not force the screams from my throat. Years of being in an abusive relationship and of avoiding the truth had created a void that sucked away my dignity and my self-defense mechanisms. I opened up and welcomed the flashbacks and pain that came to me, knowing that—as much as I hated it—I would become stronger if I could get those feelings out of the dark, out of hiding.

Samwise stood by me during those difficult times. When I was overwhelmed by painful memories, he waited for me to tell him what I needed from him. He let me cry, let me rage, let me vent, and my silent crying began to take on a voice.

And then, eventually, the pain began to lessen. The more I talked about my experiences, the less power they held over me. The more I spoke up when something bothered me, the more power I felt over my life. When I could finally shout "NO!" and mean it, I knew that I could stand up for myself, that I was less likely to become a victim again because I believed in my right to freedom from abuse.

I went through a period of rage, but over time those feelings have become manageable. I am undoubtedly more cautious than someone who's never been raped. I look in the backseat of my car before I unlock the door and get in. I carry my keys jammed between my knuckles when I'm walking down a dark street. I assess the danger quotient of an area that I am entering. I walk with my head held up and with a sturdy step because I refuse to present a would-be attacker with a willing victim.

Because of my ability to survive and come through trauma and years of insecurity, I am outspoken and nonapologetic for my stance on life's issues.

I've learned, as one friend put it, to only apologize for those things that I've personally done or said that might hurt someone.

Trauma can make a person strong; we incorporate everything that happens to us into our lives. We cannot ignore and repress events without taking on tremendous baggage.

When life gives you lemons, you make lemonade. If somebody hurts you, you take that pain and use it as fuel to make yourself stronger. Don't let the other guy win. Prove you can come out more radiant and brilliant than ever before.

A Definition of Rape

Rape is not sex. Rape uses sex as a weapon. It's a crime of violence and control. When a stranger jumps out of the bushes and hauls you down with a knife at your throat and has sex with you, that's rape. When your date overpowers you and forces you to have sex after you've been necking a while but you've said you want to stop, that's rape. When you are coerced into unwanted oral sex, even if you're not penetrated vaginally, that's rape. When someone forcibly uses an object in your vagina against your wishes, that's rape. When somebody threatens your life or the life of a loved one in order to demand sex with you, that's rape. When your husband wants sex and won't take no for an answer, that's rape. When a man is forced into sodomy or oral sex, that's rape.

States have different legal definitions for the term rape but for our purposes, we will define rape as any forcible sexual act where no consent was given.

What Rape Isn't

Rape is not consensual BDSM. Rape is not having sex with someone then regretting it the next day and accusing your partner of forcing you. Rape is not having a homosexual encounter, feeling guilty, and accusing your lover of force. While ogling and catcalls may be frustrating or even humiliating, they aren't rape. To call them that lessens the impact of true rape.

Who Are the Rape Victims and Survivors?

They are your eighty-year-old grandmother. Your three-your-old daughter. Your sister who weighs three hundred pounds. Your anorexic mother. Your little brother. Your fifty-year-old economics teacher. Your best buddy who goes fishing with you every week during trout season. Your son's track coach.

You.

Got it? Anybody can be a victim, though women are by far the most common targets. However, I personally know at least three men who've been raped. I also know a number of men who were victims of sexual assault when they were young. Estimates say between one out of three to one out of seven people will be the victim of some sexual assault during their lives.

Got it? Women, men, children; it can be anyone.

Profile of a Rapist

There is none, though most rapists are male. Rapists are

- ❧ white, black, Hispanic, Asian, Native American

- ❧ fifteen, twenty, thirty, fifty, sixty, seventy years old

- ❧ doctors, lawyers, bricklayers, unemployed, teachers, artists, cashiers, soldiers

- ❧ single, married, engaged, divorced

- parents, "a good family man," and childless, "a loner who hates children"

- friends, strangers

Are you starting to get the picture? There is no clear-cut definition. The "beware of strangers and you'll be okay" axiom no longer applies, since over half of rape victims know their attacker.

Rapists tend to repeat their crimes; chances are you won't be his only target. Unfortunately, he'll probably get away with it; over 50 percent of rapes go unreported, and of the ones that are reported, only a fraction of the criminals are caught and punished. And punishment may be a simple slap on the wrist to a few years in jail. In a number of Latin American countries, the rapist may willingly marry the victim (with or without her consent) and avoid any conviction for his crime, a throwback to Biblical injunctions that promote such a punishment.

Women are still sometimes treated as property to be bought and sold by men—another reason for my extreme position on the punishment for rapists. Not only do these monsters give a bad name to men who would never think of hurting a woman, but their accepted presence condones this attitude in their sons who grow up watching the way they treat the women in their lives. Do not doubt that if you are in an abusive situation, your daughters will grow up thinking that it's okay to be beat up and molested. Your sons will grow up believing that it's okay to molest women. You owe it to them, if not to yourself, to get out of that situation.

Prevention: The Best Medicine

There are some basic steps you can take to avoid rape. Nothing can guarantee your safety, but prevention can help you avoid becoming some psycho's toy.

Avoid dark streets at night when possible. Avoid taking shortcuts through alleys. If you have to walk down an empty street, carry your keys with the tips poking between your knuckles so, if you're attacked, you can thrust the tips of the keys in your attacker's eyes.

If you can't avoid walking through dark areas alone, carry a walking stick and learn how to use it. Walk with your head high, your step firm, and the feeling inside that if anybody fucks with you, you'll bash their brains out. Others can sense your attitude, trust me.

I used to carry a walking stick when I lived in my bus at the back of an isolated five acres of wooded land. At that time, I also used to wear a lot of face paint. One day a guy on the street approached me, but he kept his distance, and he smiled and asked, "Uh, I was wondering whether those are real tattoos on your face?" I told him no. He nodded, then said, "I bet people give you a wide berth because of that and your stick, don't they?" I gave him a big grin and said, "You got it, and that's why I carry it." Strength and confidence are not only beautiful, they inspire respect.

Don't go home (to your home or his) with any stranger. Don't give out your address to someone you don't know. If you have to meet someone at your house and you aren't sure about them, make certain that a friend knows when and where you are meeting this person. Have your friend call while your visitor is there, and set up a code to use if something is amiss. I've used this trick when new tarot clients came to my house and my husband was at work. However, I scheduled all appointments with new male clients when Samwise was going to be home.

Never leave your drink unattended in a bar, and if you accept a drink from someone you don't know, make sure you see the bartender pour it and have it handed directly to you. Ecstasy and other drugs like it are the date rapist's best friend, and you might not remember an attack for days, weeks, or months.

Lock your doors and windows at night. If it's hot, buy a fan or air conditioner and learn to sleep naked under a cool sheet. Lock your car door.

Don't spend time at the door (either car or home) fumbling for your keys; have them ready when you need them.

Hitchhiking may have been the way to get around in the '60s and '70s, but no more. I finally quit hitching when a good friend got raped on her way home from the grocery store. Don't pick up hitchhikers and don't hitch. Don't even pick up a woman; she may have a partner waiting in the bushes. Don't put yourself in danger. Don't stop unless it's clear that she's alone. Even then, she might have a gun and designs on your money.

When approached by a stranger in a parking lot, do not stay around to talk to the person. Head for a store. Too many people—women, children, and men—have been abducted from parking lots. Park in well-lit areas. If your car breaks down, raise the hood and tie a piece of material to it, turn on the emergency lights, lock the doors, and stay inside. Wait for someone to stop and offer help, then ask them to call the police or a garage for you. If you have one, keep a cell phone in your car for emergencies.

Never believe anybody who comes up to you in a mall or on the street and says, "I can make you a star" or "I can make you a model." If you have reason to think they might be telling the truth, ask for their card and say you'll give them a call. Then leave and thoroughly check them out before you call them. If their story seems bogus, talk to the cops and provide a description of the person who approached you.

If You Are Attacked

What do you do if the unthinkable happens, and you find yourself at the mercy of an attacker?

First, try to remain calm. Panic will only make an attack worse. It's hard, but you must maintain clarity so you can ascertain whether or not your life is in danger. If you avoid upsetting the rapist, you stand a better chance of walking away from the attack.

Second, remember that your goal is to stay alive. This means doing whatever you must to survive. If this means giving in to the rape and walking away with your life, then submit. If this means fighting back because you believe your attacker is going to kill you, then fight. Rely on your instincts and watch for any signals from your attacker.

If you can get the rapist to talk to you, you begin to seem more like a person and less like an object and this will, at times, lessen the aggression. Rapists often see women as objects rather than as people. When they begin to realize that you are a person, they have a harder time hurting you. If you tell the attacker you have AIDS or are pregnant, they might let you go. Some women have gotten away by doing something that disgusts the rapist, such as drooling and picking their nose or acting like they are crazy.

If you are in an enclosed environment and you scream for help, yell "Fire!" People react far more to that cry than to a cry of "Rape." If you are outside, give a piercing shriek for as long as you can or scream "9-1-1" over and over; this will usually capture attention.

Unfortunately, some psychos thrive on terrorizing their victims, getting a thrill out of the kill. In this situation, your only chance is to fight as hard and as dirty as you can. It's better to take a knife wound or a gunshot wound and survive than to be tortured and murdered.

If you have to fight, don't be afraid to go for the eyes. If somebody is attacking you, they deserve whatever they get. Too many women lose their lives because they're afraid to fight dirty. Anything goes if somebody's trying to hurt you. Go for the areas that are tender: eyes, balls, solar plexus, nose. Spiked heels can ram right through someone's foot if you stomp hard enough. Use your fingernails to rip at their face. Anything and everything can be a weapon if you use it right. Sticks on the ground work as clubs. You can throw a blanket over them while you run. Spray hairspray in their eyes and nose. Whip your backpack or purse around and smack them in the head with it. Pointy rings can damage eyes and face when scraped across the skin. Sound gruesome? It would be even more gruesome to end up on a slab at the morgue. I know. For one of my jobs, I was responsible for microfilming court cases, and I'll never forget the picture I had to film of a little girl who had been raped and strangled. The sight of her lying on that cold gray slab haunts me to this day.

Try to remember as much as you can about your attacker's looks and manner of speech. I know this is asking a lot, but it's important if you report the rape so you can help police identify him.

I've Been Raped, What Do I Do Now?

First, get yourself to someplace safe and lock your door. Call a close friend, a loved one, someone to be with you.

Right away—before you shower, before you change clothes—you have to decide whether or not you are going to report this. If I was raped today, I'd call the cops. Things were very different when I was seventeen; now law enforcement officials are given sensitivity training to help rape victims. You may wish to call a rape crisis hotline before you call the police.

If you decide to report the crime, you will need to give the police the clothing you were wearing so they can search for any DNA evidence the attacker might have left. You will also have to go to a hospital and have a gynecological exam so they can check for semen samples. You should do this anyway, and tell the doctor you were raped so they can test you for STDs, give you a morning-after pill to prevent pregnancy, and test for the HIV virus. There are some laws that provide compensation for medical expenses if you report your crime. Check with your law enforcement offices for further information.

Have someone take pictures (and document the time and date) of any bruises, cuts, and other physical damage that the rapist inflicted, for use in court as evidence. Weeks, months, sometimes even years can go by before a suspect is caught, jailed, and goes to trial. The jury will need to see what shape you were in at the time of the crime, not at the time of the trial.

Contact a lawyer. If you don't know who to call, ask the hospital's rape counselor for advice. The counselor, your lawyer, and the police should be able to adequately prepare you for what will come in court.

If you decide not to report the crime, I urge you to reconsider—he will continue to rape until he is stopped; every bit of evidence will help the police find him. If you don't want to call the cops, you should at least call a rape counseling center. They work confidentially, and they will help you over the initial trauma and will help your loved ones understand how to cope with your assault.

Tori Amos, the musician, started a foundation called RAINN—Rape, Abuse, and Incest National Network. A victim of violent rape herself, she organized this nationwide coalition to help rape, incest, and abuse victims. All calls are confidential. You can call them twenty-four hours a day, and they will link you up with someone in your area specifically trained to help rape victims. The phone number for that organization is: 1-800-656-HOPE (1-800-656-4673). The website is http://www.rainn.org.

Treat yourself very gently for as long as you need to heal. You have just survived a traumatic ordeal, be kind to yourself. Remember:

> You didn't cause it.

> You are not at fault.

> Women of all ages, shapes, and colors get raped.

> Men get raped too; this doesn't mean you aren't still strong and masculine.

> Not all men are rapists, and not all men want to hurt you.

> There's over a 60 percent chance that you will know your attacker. Your attacker may be a member of your own family. Blood ties do not give anyone a right to harm you. You owe it to yourself to stop them from doing this again.

🙵 Rape doesn't mean you are a bad person, that you failed at anything, or that you are dirty. You did not deserve what happened to you. You don't blame a five-year-old who's been molested for what happened to her, do you? Don't blame yourself. Just because you let down your guard doesn't mean that it's okay for someone else to take advantage of you. And sometimes, no matter how many precautions we take, we get trapped.

Emotions after Being Raped

What can you expect to feel the first few weeks after being raped? There are a number of reactions, and you may experience some, all, or none of them. Among the most common are

Numbness. You may feel nothing for a while, as if your body and mind are on autopilot. This is a self-defense mechanism that makes it possible to get through trauma to a time when you are ready to face your feelings again. Unfortunately, some people believe that if they feel numb, it means they weren't affected by what happened. They repress any upsurge in emotion to stay clear of what happened.

When this is done for too long, the feelings will well up, as if behind a dam, and someday they will spill over. Blocked emotions can cause you to act in ways you normally wouldn't, and they can affect your relationships and the way you interact with others if you don't address them. They can also affect your health and how you react to your sexuality and your body.

Anger. You will undoubtedly experience a lot of anger, toward your rapist and, unfortunately, toward yourself. It's perfectly natural to beat yourself up, wondering, "How could I have stopped this?" Most likely, there was nothing you could have done to prevent the assault, and even if there was, it's too late. Nobody has a right to rape or sexually assault you, regardless of how you both behaved.

Anger is part of the healing process. It's okay to be angry; it's okay to shout, to scream, to lose your temper. Sometimes it helps to beat on a pillow or a punching bag. One woman I knew had her husband build her a small enclosure where she could smash bottles onto a bed of rocks. Finding a physical outlet for your anger is a good thing; it will help lower your blood pressure and get the emotions outside your body. But don't misplace your anger; don't turn it on someone who doesn't deserve it, including yourself.

Humiliation. Unfortunately, one of the emotions we have to deal with when we've been assaulted is a feeling of humiliation. We have been violated, exposed, and used against our will. This is a hard one; recovering your dignity will require work and time. Remember that they can assault your body and strip you of every shred of self-control, but they cannot touch your inner core that makes you "you." No matter what they've done, they can't own your heart and soul; that is yours, forever.

There are a few people who were tortured and traumatized in childhood to such a degree that they developed multiple personalities just to be able to survive the abuse. Their injuries, both emotional and physical, were so bad that it shattered their sense of self before it had a chance to fully develop. Some of them, once the problem is identified, may be able to integrate back into a fully functional state.

Guilt. We may feel guilty after the attack. We may be blaming ourselves for bringing it on or not preventing it. If only we hadn't been walking down that street . . . if only we had looked before we got into the car . . . if only we hadn't trusted our friend's friend. The important thing to remember here is: we did not cause the attack; we are not responsible for our attacker's actions.

Guilt might also creep in in memory of the fact that, while rape is never something we want, our bodies might seem to have betrayed us. Sexual response can be heightened by adrenaline, and some victims might have an orgasm during an attack. They feel doubly guilty; they were attacked, and they had a pleasurable response at one point. Don't beat yourself up over this. It happens, and it doesn't mean that you deserved or wanted the attack; it doesn't mean that you are a bad person.

Other reactions include

- ❧ a feeling that you have lost your boundaries. This is common for survivors of any attack. Your body has been imposed on, and you need to reclaim your space and cleanse your aura.

- ❧ nightmares and sleeplessness. I still have nightmares, years later, but they have evolved over the past five years or so. Now, in my nightmares where I'm being attacked, I fight back; I say "no" and I stop the attack. For sleeplessness, try soothing baths and herbal teas. Use sleeping pills only as directed by your doctor and only for limited periods of time. You don't need a drug dependency on top of everything else.

- ❧ trouble coping with well-meaning but uninformed friends. There's nothing quite like the friend who says, "But it's been three weeks. You should be over it by now." Tell these people that you are dealing with the situation the best way you know how, that you thank them for their concern, but that you trust your counselor and his or her wisdom.

Evolving from a Victim to a Survivor

At some point, you need to evolve from a victim to a survivor. If you stay in the victim mentality, you run the risk of shutting down your entire life and putting it on hold, of developing unhealthy patterns for relationships and behavior, and of losing your personal power. Your attacker disrupted your life once; do you want to give him control over how you live the rest of your life? Do you want to give him the power to affect you the rest of your days? Until you can let go of being a victim, that's exactly what you are doing.

It isn't easy, it takes a lot of time and work, but it's worth it to reclaim your sense of self-control. I recommend that you talk to a rape crisis counselor. For me, having the freedom to talk my pain out helped me heal. Sam was the first man I'd been with who encouraged me to get angry when I was angry. He wanted me to shout, to scream if necessary, to express my feelings. And by learning to get angry, by not keeping my feelings inside, I was able to let go of those lingering feelings of anger, humiliation, and guilt, one by one.

I established boundaries of what is and is not okay. I don't like to be hugged by strangers, even readers who really want to reach out and give me a hug. Sometimes I acquiesce and sometimes I don't, depending on the person. It's not that I don't want to be friendly, but I do not want my boundaries violated without my permission.

By the same token, I staunchly defend allowing children *not* to be forced into hugging their parent's friends or other family members if they don't want to. Maybe they sense something about Uncle John that makes them uncomfortable. Maybe Aunt Mary kisses them a bit too firmly on the lips. Maybe it's all innocent, but children have a right to own their bodies. When you demand that someone allow themselves to be touched by strangers when they don't want to, you set up a pattern. You condition them to believe that they don't have a right to say "I don't want to be touched/kissed/hugged/fucked."

I also gave myself permission not to forgive my attacker. I find both opposition to and agreement with my stance, but I stick by it. I don't believe you have to forgive your attacker. I have no interest in loving the perverts of this world, and all the white light in the universe ain't gonna do most of them any good. I want to expend my energy on those I can help empower, whom I can help recover, whom I can help learn to love themselves and their world.

It's true that hate uses up a lot of energy. Though I don't forgive my attacker, I don't waste energy on hating him anymore. He doesn't deserve even that much of my attention. In fact, writing this chapter was the first time in ages that I've really thought about that night, and the only reason I'm going into it is to try and help those who've been attacked and don't know what to do. I'm being open with my experience to let you know that you are not alone. This happens to a lot of people.

When you are comfortable with the idea, you will want to work with the chapter on masturbation to reclaim your sexual emotions and boundaries. You need to feel love for your genitals, for your body. It's not your fault that you were attacked, and you shouldn't treat your sexuality as the culprit. Go slow; learn to enjoy the feeling of your hands on your body again. The joys of your body will shine through the damage done to you. You can reclaim your sense of pride, of self, and of sensuality. You might also want to work with the ritual at the end of this chapter to help you on a magical level. It's geared toward a group but can be adapted for solitary work if you prefer that.

There will come a day when you will be able to look back on the attack and remember it without getting swept up in the fear and anguish. You will be able to say, "Yes it happened, but it did not defeat me. I survived, and I am stronger than I was before." And that, my friends, is a wonderful feeling.

Everything we do, everything we feel and think and experience, makes us who we are in the present, and the present is constantly evolving. You can turn terror into strength, humiliation into dignity, and take pride in who you are today.

Special Circumstances: A Note to Minors

A sexual assault can disrupt your entire life. If someone fondles you on the breasts, penis, vagina, or anywhere else on your genitals, that is considered sexual abuse, or molestation, and you should tell a trusted adult. If you are a minor and are the victim of incest, if your father, mother, brother, uncle, stepfather, sister, aunt, grandfather, grandmother, or cousin sexually assaults you, you *must* tell someone. If an adult who is not related to you assaults you—you *must* tell someone.

If you don't think your immediate family will be supportive, then talk to a trusted teacher, a school counselor, or a rape crisis center. If one person doesn't listen to you, talk to another and another until you find someone who does. You can always call 1-800-656-HOPE (1-800-656-4673), and the people there will help you find someone to talk to. Their website is www.rainn.org, and they can help you sort through what needs to happen next and help you find counseling.

No matter what happens, please don't think that you are a bad person. If, for example, your father molested you and you turn him in, your mother may not be as supportive as you hope. She is probably in shock. Ideally she will protect you, support you, and do what needs to be done. She is probably confused and mixed up, and it may take some time before she fully understands what happened. Your brothers and sisters may have been abused too, and they might be afraid to say anything. If you have seen that your siblings were abused, you need to tell someone. No matter what, nobody has a right to sexually abuse you.

If you were molested, you may experience feelings of confusion. Your body may enjoy some of the sensations that happen during the attack, even when you are afraid and upset. Don't feel guilty about this; it is a normal reaction.

You may also find yourself angry and acting out toward others. This is also natural. We try to maintain control in our lives where we can, and sometimes the only way we feel strong when we've been hurt is by hurting others. This doesn't mean the behavior is appropriate, however, and you should talk to your counselor about it. Once you have worked through your feelings of betrayal and anger, your temper will probably calm down.

You might find that you still love the person who abused you. This is also normal. We have mixed feelings when family members hurt us, and it's hard to reconcile those feelings. Sometimes we just have to accept that people we love can and do hurt us. But they should be stopped before they hurt somebody else, and they must accept their punishment for what they've done.

Adults know better than to hurt children; no excuse can make their actions right. You did not cause them to do what they did, nor did you tempt them; and their actions are *their* responsibility.

Never lie and say someone molested or raped you when they didn't. You are bound to be found out, and you will cause pain for yourself as well as those around you. If you are Pagan, remember that we must accept responsibility for what we say and do. Lying about something like this affects your karma and may plague you the rest of your life.

If someone has touched you and made you uncomfortable, and you don't know whether or not what they did is considered abuse, ease your mind by calling the number I gave previously, and talk to a counselor who can help you sort out your feelings on the subject and advise you. Anytime that someone touches you in a suggestive manner and you don't like it, tell them to stop.

A Note for Partners and Families of Sexual Assault Victims

Whether your partner was raped by a stranger, a friend, or a family member, you have a special role to fulfill in his or her healing. But it is important to remember that your loved one will need to go at their own pace.

If you've never been through it, you can't possibly understand the depths to which emotions can sink when you're fighting for self-recovery. Having your body violated in this innermost manner is both terrifying and infuriating. The survivor's anger can be incredible, and their fear can be overwhelming.

> ❧ Watch your ego. If you react as if she's your possession and that the assault on her was an insult to you, you are only reinforcing

the idea that she doesn't have a right to her own body and her own anger. She won't have the energy to help you handle your feelings of confusion right now. She needs your support and strength, not a punctured ego to deal with.

- Get counseling for yourself if you feel her needs are overwhelming you. Encourage her to get counseling.

- If you are lovers, expect that your sex life will be disrupted for some time, and don't be angry with her about this. Masturbate while alone; don't make her feel guilty, and don't give her an ultimatum. If her sexual resistance keeps up, quietly insist that the two of you visit a counselor together. It may take weeks or even months before she's ready to have sex again.

- Keep it foremost in your mind that she did not cause this assault, that it is not her fault. Do not blame her or suggest ways in which she might have avoided it. Men tend to try and solve problems rather than just listening and being supportive. She doesn't need to hear that you think she could have walked down a different street or that she could have had her keys ready when she got to the car. She needs you to listen to her fear, her anger, her worries, and her pain.

- If she wants to prosecute her attacker, support her in whatever ways you can. A court case is traumatic, and she'll need your encouragement to give her strength.

- Don't overprotect her or you'll run the risk of smothering her. She needs encouragement to face the world again in her own time, and there's no way you can guarantee her lifelong safety.

- Don't go into a macho rage and rant about how you will "get this bastard" who hurt her; your anger may intensify her fear and feelings of guilt.

- Encourage her to take a martial arts class, and go with her if she wants you to. Don't get angry if she spends time at a support group for survivors; she's trying to heal. On the other hand, the healing process can get bogged down; for a few victims, the support groups feel so safe that they don't want to move on. If you think she's stuck, talk to her about it, and if you need to, talk to her counselor about it.

- When she is ready to have sex again, take it slow; let her take the lead. Ask her what she wants, how she would like you to proceed. If she resists a particular position or activity, don't press it. Her attacker may have forced her into oral sex or sodomy, for example, and she will have to come to terms with those particular acts in her own time. She may want either less or more sex than before. Discuss your evolving relationship with each other and, if necessary, with a counselor.

- When the victim is a man, he will have special needs of his own to deal with; feelings of emasculation are common. Don't ever joke about the attack or question his sexuality or his masculinity. Offer your support as you would for a woman. Encourage him to get counseling, and offer to go with him if he wants that. Men are often reluctant to get counseling for this problem.

- When the victim is a child, do whatever you can to make them feel safe. Encourage them to talk about the assault, even if it's hard for you to listen. Make sure they know that you don't blame them for what happened, and keep an eye out for any signs of inappropriate acting out. Get them to a counselor. Enroll them into a children's tai chi or karate class so they feel empowered. Report the adult who abused them, whether or not it's a family member or close friend. Do not trust that this is an isolated incident. Most pedophiles are repeat offenders.

As the loved one of a sexual assault victim, you will play a vital role in their healing, but do not forget to attend to your own needs. If you need counseling, get it. If you don't think you can handle some of the problems that come up, be honest and tell your partner that you can't be her sole support system. When a family member is raped, be it wife, child, sibling, or husband, it affects the whole family. We are not individuals who drift on the tides, isolated and alone. We must be there for each other.

Ceremony of Persephone: A Reclamation of Power for Women Who've Been Attacked

There are times in our lives when we look to ritual and magic to reclaim, purify, and balance our sexual selves. This ritual is not meant to replace counseling for assault victims; in fact, it will not help if you aren't ready. Magic is not a substitute for all the emotional work that we need to do.

This ritual is for someone who is ready to leave behind their intense fear after an attack, and their wishes should always be respected. If, partway through, they don't think they can go through with it, if they are still too wrapped in the pain, then quietly open the Circle and spend the afternoon talking and chatting. Never pressure an assault victim into moving faster than she can truly handle. We have to go outside our comfort zones to heal, but not before we are ready.

Note: This ceremony is woman centered, with no male energy involved since a vast majority of those assaulted are female. Men should consult a Pagan priest to devise an appropriate ritual. If you like, you may alter this one for gender differences. Most men I know who've been assaulted have been very close-mouthed about it, and I don't know whether a group ritual would be effective or comfortable for them, though this may be due to social pressures and the stigma attached to men who've been raped and molested.

Please note, this ritual is a long one. The women involved must be dedicated to seeing the entire process through. Allow a complete afternoon or a full evening in which to do this, and don't make any plans for afterward so nobody feels rushed. The ritual is complex, though simple if you examine the elements separately. The goal is to cleanse your body and soul after an assault. An assault can leave you feeling dirty. Violation creates great turmoil in the aura, and if we can calm and cleanse our energy, then we can speed healing and recovery. This ritual can also help reclaim a sense of boundaries.

Gather close friends who will be supportive and understanding. The ideal group size is from five to ten women. Too many people diffuses the focus. As always, adapt the ritual as necessary to meet your special circumstances and needs.

It would be wonderful for this ritual if you had access to a swimming pool or a secluded (and safe) pool of water in nature, in which case you should alter the ceremony to fit the circumstances. Obviously, you won't be pouring artificial soap and salts into a stream of running water, but you can use lavender and rose waters to splash on yourself during the immersion. Barring that, you need a bathtub or hot tub filled with lukewarm water. You will be changing the water partway through the ritual so don't use up all the warm water at the start.

For the first part of the ritual, you will need

▷ lavender bath salts

▷ a sage smudge stick or purifying incense

- pomegranate juice (to drink)

- a magical Protection Oil (if you don't have this, substitute rosemary, rose geranium, or a protective essential oil)

- a ritual broom for each member of the Circle

- a black candle

For the second part of the ritual, you will need

- rose bath salts

- rose incense

- apple juice or apple cider (to drink)

- Strength Oil (the recipe is given at the end of the chapter; if you don't have this, substitute dragon's blood oil or High John the Conqueror Oil)

- a red candle

- cakes and wine

Set the altar with a white, black, and red cloth—the colors of the Goddess. You may, if you like, drape it with pearls, shells, pine cones, and other objects that represent the healing aspects of nature.

In this ritual, we will refer to the woman who was attacked as the survivor.

Designate one woman to be the Priestess—probably the most experienced or the one to whom the survivor feels closest—and one woman to be her assistant. Begin by asking the assistant to fill the tub and sprinkle lavender bath salts under the running water.

When the bath is ready, the assistant should smudge all the areas where the ritual will take place, such as the bath and the living room. She should then gather the women to one side as the Priestess casts a Circle. Each woman except the survivor should have a ritual broom with her. After casting the Circle, the Priestess should invoke the elements.

Turn to the north, and say:

Spirit of the Earth, Spirit of foundations and stability, come to this Circle and bring with you your strength and your ever-evolving sense of growth, that you might create a new foundation upon which we may rest, a platform of solidity where we might once again find our center of balance. Welcome, Spirit of the Earth, and Blessed Be.

Turn to the east, and say:

Spirit of the Wind, Spirit of new beginnings, come to this Circle and bring with you your cleansing and purifying breezes, that you might sweep through to clear away stagnation and old hurts and open the gate for new clarity and inner peace. Welcome, Spirit of the Wind, and Blessed Be.

Turn to the south, and say:

Spirit of the Flame, Spirit of transmutation, come to this Circle and bring with you your fires that destroy outworn and unneeded energy, that you might burn through and leave, under the ashes, a new sense of sexuality, creativity, and personal power. Welcome, Spirit of the Flame, and Blessed Be.

Turn to the west, and say:

Spirits of the Waves, Spirit of the Ocean Mother who encircles this planet in her embrace, come to this Circle and bring with you tears of sorrow and tears of joy. Flow through our psyches, heal the wounds of violation, and transform stagnant and murky waters into forceful

rivers of clarity. Let us glimpse the hidden depths of our beings.
Welcome, Spirits of the Waves, and Blessed Be.

Then the Priestess will invoke the goddess Persephone:

Brilliant and terrible, compassionate and sweet, Persephone, Queen of
the Underworld, I call to you—you who understand the nature of viola-
tion, Goddess you are, who yourself has been abducted and raped. Come
to us as the nurturing queen, compassionate Lady, survivor of pain. Be
with us in our rites as we offer (name of woman assaulted) our
strength, love, and support in order that she might heal and reclaim her
own sense of self, even as you transmuted your own pain into power.
Wise Persephone, daughter of Demeter, Welcome and Blessed Be."

As each woman enters the circle, the assistant will smudge her and say:

Enter this Circle in love and trust. Be safe here, and offer safety here.
Be loved here, and offer love. Join us under the eyes of the Goddess, and
feel her embrace as you enter her sacred space.

As each woman enters the Circle and comes to her place, she will lay her
broom down by her feet. The woman who was attacked should enter the
Circle last, and she will not be smudged until later. Before the survivor
enters, the priestess will ask her a series of questions that she must answer
honestly. If she answers "no" to any of the questions, the ritual should stop;
she isn't ready to go through the ritual at this time. The Priestess will ask:

&ediexclaim; Have you asked for help in your healing and received it?

&ediexclaim; Have you accepted that you were attacked, that you will forever be
changed, but that you can grow, evolve, and strengthen from this?

&ediexclaim; Do you understand that the process of reclaiming your boundaries
will take time, and is never easy? That you may find yourself
backsliding into fear at times, and that this is normal?

⤷ Can you honestly say that you are ready to move out of your pain, that you have reached the point where you can start to let it go, let it be?

If she answers yes to all four questions, she will be invited to enter the Circle. The Priestess should say:

Enter this Circle in love and trust. Be safe here, and offer safety here. Be loved here, and offer love. Join us under the eyes of the Goddess and feel her embrace as you enter her sacred space.

The survivor should walk around the Circle deosil (clockwise), and each member will give her a light hug or a kiss as she passes to show support. This may bring her to tears, which is okay; crying is part of the healing process. After the survivor has made her way around the Circle, the Priestess should lead her to the center. The women around the Circle should join hands to create a tight ring of energy. The Priestess says:

We can never help you become as you were before, for there is no going back. But we can help you cleanse your energy and remove lingering traces of the assailant's energy from your aura. We can support you as you reclaim your boundaries and power from the person who hurt you. Remove your clothes, to stand naked and beautiful and strong in the light of the Goddess.

The Priestess should help the survivor remove her clothes. The survivor may feel very exposed, but she should try to persevere. Feelings of vulnerability are natural after an attack, and a woman-only ritual can help ease them. If the participants feel comfortable, they can work skyclad to support their friend.

Once the survivor is naked, the assistant will slowly smudge her and say:

By the purifying tendrils of sage and cedar (or whatever incense you are using), let your energy be cleansed. Let this sacred smoke filter through your aura and remove all unwanted energies, all unwelcome visitors and lingering fears. Breathe deep the smoke of the Goddess, and know she is in your lungs, embracing you, cleansing and purifying your body, mind, and spirit.

Next, the Priestess will light the black candle on the altar. The assistant will offer the survivor the glass of pomegranate juice to drink, and she says:

As so Persephone was destined to walk into the Underworld, so have you been forced to journey deep into pain. Drink of the pomegranate now to signify that you live in balance, between light and dark, and that you can return from the shadows and blossom again.

After the survivor has drained the goblet, the Priestess will open a gateway in the Circle to the east:

I create a gateway that is protected from all things unwelcome.

The Priestess then takes her ritual broom and begins to sweep the woman's aura. (Be careful not to hit her with the broom; it won't hurt her if you accidentally brush her, but broom bristles are never much fun along bare skin.) As the Priestess sweeps the offending energy off of the woman's aura, everyone envisions her fear and anger and worry being swept away. The survivor should focus on releasing these things from her heart and her body. The women forming the Circle should drop hands and use their brooms to help sweep the energy widdershins around the Circle, forming a counterclockwise spiral from the Priestess out. Each woman will be picking up the energy from the person on her left and sweeping it to the person on her right, from the center (the Priestess) to the northeast, around the circle and out through the gateway at the east.

Once the negative energy is swept out of the Circle, the assistant uses the Protection Oil to anoint her own forehead, then the forehead of the woman next to her, who then anoints the woman on her right and so on. Do this in a widdershins direction. The oil should come last to the Priestess, who will anoint the survivor.

The Priestess now takes the black candle and leads the survivor into the bath, where she will bathe in the lavender-scented water to calm her aura and wash away any lingering residue.

During this time, the women in the main room will prepare the altar with the red candle, the Strength Oil, a goblet of apple juice, and the rose incense. The cakes and wine should be ready, but they don't have to be on the altar.

When the survivor dries off, the Priestess will lead her back into the room and through the gateway. The assistant will leave the Circle to empty the bathtub and refill it with clean water and rose bath salts. While she is gone, the women can relax on the floor; it would be nice to have plenty of cushions and soft throws around for everyone to sit on. When the assistant returns, the Priestess will light the red candle and say:

Red is the color of strength, the color of our blood, the color of our power. Those who have survived rape and attack are, in truth, warriors of the highest kind, Amazons who refuse to be bested, who refuse to hate all for the actions of one. We celebrate and invoke our strength, our power, and our sexuality, as it surges from the very core of the divine feminine into our bodies and our souls. We do not freeze, go into hiding, or retire from the world, but go out boldly, heads held high, refusing to capitulate to fear and anger. We use our pain and anger as fuel, transforming them into our art, our good works, our strength.

The Priestess gives survivor the bottle of Strength Oil. She anoints her own forehead and says:

I reclaim my power. I reclaim my strength. What was broken, I mend. What was scarred is now stronger, for scar tissue is always stronger

than unblemished flesh. I set my boundaries, and I insist that others
abide by them. I invoke the strength of Persephone into my life.

She hands the oil to the Priestess, who anoints her own forehead and repeats the above, the passes the bottle deosil around the Circle, each woman following suit. When every woman has anointed herself, the assistant will hand the apple juice to the survivor, who drains the goblet as the Priestess says:

Drink of the apple of strength and beauty, and know that it grows
within you and shines through your eyes and your smile.

The assistant will then smudge each person with the rose incense (the Priestess should smudge the assistant first), saying:

Within strength is beauty, and every rose has thorns that may prick
and rip if one is not careful. We celebrate our thorns even as we
celebrate our beauty.

After the smudging, each woman should step forward and, in turn, briefly tell of a moment in her life when she overcame an attack or a fear. Everything that is said must be true.

For example, one might say:

I survived being beaten by my ex-husband. I've grown strong, and the
fear of his anger no longer affects me. So mote it be.

After the survivor has spoken, and she should go last, the Priestess will take the red candle and lead her through the gateway to the bath. Now she will bathe in the strength and beauty of roses. The women in the main room can use this time to talk about their own experiences, while staying positive and focused on healing, or to meditate on their own lives.

When the survivor and the Priestess return, the assistant will pass around cakes and wine, and toasts should be made to the Goddess. At this point, the Priestess will devoke the elements, bid farewell to Persephone, then open the Circle. A potluck dinner is a good follow-up to return to the mundane. It's very important to ground after this ritual, for it is a long one, and it's important to get a breath of fresh air and clear out the energy in the house. In fact, if it's warm enough you might wish to throw open the doors and windows and let the breeze sweep through to cleanse the space.

Strength Oil

This oil is exceptionally good for self-empowerment spells.

$^{1}/_{4}$ ounce olive oil
9 drops lime oil
9 drops orange oil
9 drops frankincense oil
9 drops dragon's blood oil
2 drops cinnamon oil
5 drops rose geranium oil
flowers: orange blossoms or frankincense resin
gems: carnelian or garnet

CHAPTER ELEVEN
The Divine
Nature of Sex

Phebe: Good shepherd, tell this youth what 'tis to love.
Silvius: It is to be all made of sighs and tears . . .
It is to be all made of faith and service . . .
It is to be all made of fantasy,
All made of passion, and all made of wishes;
All adoration, duty, and observance;
All humbleness, all patience, and impatience;
All purity, all trial, all obeisance.

WILLIAM SHAKESPEARE, *As You Like It*

The gods and goddesses of sex, passion, and lust are many in name, most having other aspects as well. Once we have tasted the delights of sexual communion, of the heights to which this form of sexuality can take us, it's hard to give that up and go back to the way we had sex before.

The following table lists some of the goddesses and gods of sex and passion, a little about their background, and corresponding gems, flowers, animals, and perfumes, if known. Where correspondences are difficult to find, I've made suggestions (which are noted by an asterisk).

The Divine Nature of Beauty

Deity and Origin	Description	Correspondences
Aphrodite: Greek goddess	Foam born of the sea, Aphrodite rules over all aspects of love, sexuality, and beauty. She is married to Hephaestus, ugly god of the forge, and often has dalliances with Ares, where we see the connection of love and hate. Venus is like a Roman Aphrodite.	Gems: emerald, turquoise Flowers: rose, clover, myrtle Animals: dove, swan, sparrow Perfumes: rose, red sandalwood
Bast: Egyptian goddess	Goddess of cats, the dance, ecstasy, and beauty, Lady Bast is often depicted as lion- or cat-headed. Her rites often include orgiastic ceremonies.	*Gems: peridot, gold, turquoise *Flowers: rose, lotus, fern Animals: cats of all kinds *Perfumes: lotus, orange, amber
Circe: Greek goddess	Goddess of seduction, magic, the Underworld, and passion, she rules over the dangers of temptation.	*Gems: garnet, obsidian Flowers: willow, fruits Animals: sows, lions, wolves *Perfumes: amber
Dionysus: Greek god	God of ecstasy, fertility, vegetation, and wine, he is the "twice born." His followers, the Maenads, partook in orgiastic ceremonies that on occasion included human sacrifice. He ruled over the Satyrs. Bacchus, the Roman god, is very similar to Dionysus.	*Gems: moonstone, garnet Flowers: grapes, ivy, vine *Animals: ram, bull, goat *Perfumes: musk, patchouli
Eros: Greek god	God of erotic love, passion, and desire, he rules both heterosexual and homosexual. Often seen as an irresponsible and chaotic deity, in actuality he rules over the complexities of how we interact in our various relationships.	*Gems: garnet, ruby, rose quartz *Flowers: rose, poppy, lotus *Perfumes: musk, rose, ylang-ylang, jasmine

Deity and Origin	Description	Correspondences
Freyja: Norse goddess	Norse goddess of beauty, sexuality, and war, she is by some accounts married to Odin, by others to another deity. Queen of the Valkyries, she has first pick over those slain in battle. She wears the sacred necklace Brisingamen.	Gems: amber, copper, turquoise Flowers: poppies, rose, cypress Animals: housecats; boar Perfumes: amber, myrrh
Freyr: Norse god	Norse god of the Vanir, he is brother to Freyja. He is lord of fertility, sensuality, abundance, joy, and beauty, among other things.	*Gems: amber, copper *Flowers: rose, cypress, Animals: boar *Perfumes: musk, patchouli
Indra: Hindu god	God of sensuality, he rules storms, thunder, lightning, passion, and many other realms.	Gems: amethyst, sapphire, lapis lazuli Flowers: shamrock, olive, aloe Animals: white elephant, horse Perfumes: cedar, saffron
Ishtar: Assyro-Babylonian goddess	Goddess of the Moon, she rules love, battle, storms, and marriage. She is connected with Inanna and Isis, and is also connected with the Hieros Gamos or Great Rite.	Gems: diamond, sapphire, ruby Flowers: olive, lily, lotus *Animals: lion, scorpion Perfumes: myrrh, dragon's blood
Kali: Hindu goddess	Goddess of destruction, passion, the fierce side of women's sexuality, and nature, she is a creatrix even through her destruction.	*Gems: carnelian, garnet, ruby Flowers: marigolds Animals: goats, sheep (especially their blood) Perfumes: spicy scents, *dragon's blood

Deity and Origin	Description	Correspondences
Lilitu: Sumerian goddess	Goddess of sexuality, she rules storms, nightmares, and demons.	*Gems: garnets, obsidian, black onyx *Flowers: narcissus, poppy, jasmine Animals: screech owl, snake *Perfumes: dark musk, peach, violet
Medhbh (Maeve): Irish goddess	Goddess of passion, she rules the faerie, battles, sexuality, and sovereignty.	*Gems: peridot, moonstone, garnet *Flowers: violet, narcissus, hyacinth *Animals: owl, raven, hind *Perfumes: lemongrass, violet, thyme
Pan: Greek god	God of passion, the woodlands, fertility, panic, and ecstasy, Pan is a satyr whose position as god of music was taken by Apollo.	Gems: black diamond Flowers: hemp, thistle Animals: goat, ass Perfumes: musk, civet
Shakti: Hindu goddess	Primordial Hindu goddess of energy, associated with Parvati, Kali, and several other Devis, she is recognized as separate and distinct. She is the feminine aspect of Shiva, without whom he cannot act.	*Gems: quartz crystal, turquoise *Flowers: willow, lily *Animals: scorpion, sphinx *Perfumes: all intoxicating scents
Shiva: Hindu god	Lord of the Dance, the Blue God, Prince of Demons, the male principle of the universe, he cannot act without Shakti. His other aspects are wed to Kali-Ma and to Parvati.	Gems: ruby, turquoise Flowers: tiger lily, geranium Animals: bull, ram, owl Perfumes: dragon's blood, musk
Yarilo: Slavonic god	God of sexuality, passion, and fertility, he is a cyclic vegetation god.	*Gems: emerald, diamond *Flowers: vine, ivy, grape *Animals: ram, bull, goat *Perfumes: musk, patchouli, cedar

If you choose to invoke one or more of these deities for ritual, please research to be certain that they are the ones you truly want to invoke. Some deities have more than one aspect; some have dark natures, and you don't want to open yourself up to an energy you will later regret.

When we meet a new partner, when we enter a new relationship, we should discuss sexuality before getting too deeply involved, before opening our bodies to a potential mate. Though love can grow out of friendship, it is more difficult to foster passion when there is no spark or chemistry. It is hard for love (in an emotional-sexual context) to flourish when the sexual connection is tenuous and the physical attraction is weak. The sexual drive will always be with us, whether found in the passion of a husband and wife, the sensuality of a woman and her lesbian lover, or the sexual play of a man and his gay partner.

Interview with Your Sexual Self

Rather than a guided meditation, I'm going to provide you with an interview for yourself, to discover more about your personal beliefs on sexuality. There are several questions each on several subjects. You might wish to work in a journal format. Take your time; there are no right or wrong answers. This will simply help you figure out where you are in terms of relating to your sexuality, where you're comfortable and where you might wish to make changes.

Youth and Sexuality

When we are young, our sexual feelings are innocent. However, that innocence can be abused by adults who give us mixed messages about sex. We may have had experiences when we were young that we remember fondly. Some were simple play; others provided lessons with long-term repercussions.

What did you think sex was about? Do you remember what you were told about sex when you were a child? Was your instruction misleading (that babies were found in the cabbage patch), or was it factual? Who told you about sex?

> ➥ After you learned about sex, what did you think it would be like when you grew up?

> ➥ When do you first remember masturbating? Were you ever caught, and if so, were you made to feel this was a bad thing to do?

> ➥ Did you ever play "doctor" with your friends? Many children have both heteroerotic and homoerotic experiences with their peers. I did, and I know many others who did. Do you think it was harmful, or was it simply an innocent childhood experience?

> ➥ What is the first sexual experience that you remember? Were you alone? What are your feelings surrounding this experience?

> ➥ If your first sexual experience was pleasurable, how do you think it contributed to your sexuality today? If your first sexual experience was traumatic, what have you done to resolve the issues it brings up in your encounters now?

Teenaged Angst

The teen years are hormonal, angst-ridden, and often the worst period of our lives. I do not understand why people insist on reinforcing the notion to young adults that these are the best years of their lives. The majority of teenagers I talk to are miserable, insecure, and in that restless, searching stage that leaves them uncertain about their existence. During this time we may have our first "knowledgeable" sexual experiences, where we fully realize what we are doing. However, at this age, we are still too young to understand that we are making a choice with an inherent responsibility. I believe this is one reason why so many teens do not use proper precautions and end up pregnant or infected with an STD.

> During your teens, your hormones went wild as you matured sexually. How did you handle this? Did you lose your virginity early or late? Did you feel left out when others talked about sex?

> Do you remember your first wet dream? How old were you when you started menstruating and what were your feelings connected to that? How did you feel when you got your first bra? Were you embarrassed, proud, anxious? Most teens are embarrassed at some point by their bodies, how did you handle these feelings?

> Some teens have periodic crushes, whether on celebrities or peers. Do you remember whom you were crazy about? (Okay, I'll admit it; when I was thirteen, I had a wild crush on Roddy McDowell, which changed the moment I laid eyes on Malcolm McDowell, then on James Earl Jones, then on David Bowie.)

Masturbation

Masturbation, at any age, is a highly personal subject. Whether practiced for pure pleasure or out of frustration, it does offer a release from pent-up sexual tensions, and it is an invaluable method of empowering ourselves. If we can bring pleasure to ourselves, if we can make ourselves feel good, then we strengthen our self-image. If we can do so without feeling guilty or embarrassed, then we will enjoy our lives on a deeper and more fulfilling level.

> How do you feel about masturbation at this point in your life? Do you masturbate now? Do you use sex toys when you do? If not, is it because you're embarrassed to pleasure yourself or to buy the sex aids, or because you simply don't feel the need?

- Has anyone (since you became an adult) caught you while you were masturbating? How did that make you feel and how did you handle it?

- Have you ever walked in on someone who was masturbating. If so, what did you do?

- Have you ever pleasured yourself in front of a partner? Was it exciting? Do you think you'd do it again? Would you like to see your partner masturbate?

Fantasy

Fantasy keeps our imaginations active. Visualization is an extension of fantasy, which is an integral part of our magic. Sexual fantasy is normal and not hurtful as long as you don't demand an unwilling partner to participate or engage in harmful activities.

- What are your favorite fantasies? Have they changed over the years or do you have some that have lingered since your younger days?

- If you have a mate, do you feel guilty about fantasizing? If you fantasize about someone else's mate, do you feel guilty about that? How do you cope with feelings of guilt?

- If you have a mate, do you ever tell them about your fantasies? If yes, how does this make you feel?

- Have you ever acted out one of your fantasies? If so, was it as pleasurable as you thought it would be? Would you like to try manifesting one of your fantasies someday, or are you content with them remaining imaginary?

Sexual Play

Sex with a partner can be sizzling, warm, cuddly, passionate, or fervid, or it can be cold, bland, boring, or angry. How we relate to our partners sexually will affect the rest of our relationship. If we have an unhappy sex life, this dissatisfaction will creep into other areas of our lives. Past relationships can help us identify any patterns of sexual problems we may have so we can avoid them in the future. As always, it's important to keep the lines of communication with ourselves and others open and clear.

- If you are sexually active, are you content with your current sex life? If you are celibate at this time, is it by choice or due to the lack of a suitable partner? How do you feel about this?

- Are there aspects to your sex life that you feel you're missing? What are they and why can't you pursue them? If they are harmless, why don't you pursue them?

- If you currently have a partner, are you upset with him or her because he or she won't try certain sexual activities that you would like to experiment with? Is your partner frustrated? If yes to either, how are you coping with this? Can you find a compromise together?

- If you currently have a partner and you're both satisfied sexually, how have you achieved this? What do you need to do to maintain this contentment?

- How many sexual partners have you had? Do you feel like you've either missed out on experience, or had too much?

- How do you feel about your gender orientation? Are you comfortable being (gay/bisexual/heterosexual)?

Think of other questions you might want to explore about your sexuality. Make this a personal journey to discover more about yourself.

Freaks 'R' Us

I'm mixing business with leather . . .
Freaks flock together . . .

BECK HANSEN, "MIXED BIZNESS," *Midnite Vultures*

Once again, I come to the end of a book. I thought that *Sexual Ecstasy & the Divine* was finished some months back, but when offered the chance to expand it fully, the challenge and opportunity was too great to pass up, and so I discovered that it was not, indeed, finished. But here it is.

No other of my nonfiction books have touched me as much as *Crafting the Body Divine* and *Sexual Ecstasy & the Divine*. They forced me to look deep within myself, to see my body, spirit, and sexuality, to overcome fears and look beyond superficialities.

I am smiling through my tears as I write this. I usually cry when I finish a book, but this time it feels as if a weight has lifted inside, a stone under which I used to hide my own fears and vulnerabilities and oddities. Now, with these books, I have rolled it away, and I'll never be able to hide under it again. The feeling is both terrifying and liberating. I think I'll grow to like it as I get used to it.

I fully expect that some folks will label me a slut or a bitch or, as one man once called me, the devil's mistress, because of the explicit and liberal nature of my work, and you know what? I will take those words, infuse them with power, and use them to fuel my inner strength.

When I sit and look at just how far out on the fringe I am, there are times when I wonder why the gods picked me for this path. I'm a Cherokee-Irish, bisexual, tattooed, fat, sensual, passionate, and brilliant Witch, who is into BDSM. I'm far from politically correct on some issues, terribly practical on most things, and comfortable calling myself a feminine feminist, while still avowing a love for both men and women. I also love collecting teapots, reading *Victoria* magazine, cooking, and keeping a lovely home. And I'm so focused on my writing and art that it's hard to get me out of my office at times.

But, like it or not, what most people see first is my freak side. So be it. If this is what it takes to get the information out there, then I will stand up and be the Freaks 'R' Us pinup girl (I like that term better than poster child). I'm willing to stand up and publicly talk about the things we've kept in the closet far too long. I will try to break media stereotypes, whichever image they may be:

- clumsy, unpopular, unattractive fat girl

- whip-wielding, PVC-clad slut

- brainy, absentminded, always-serious writer

- over-forty, married, boring housewife

- flaky, New Age, totally impractical fluff bunny, Witchy-Poo

- ascetic metaphysician totally uninterested in worldly goods

I will challenge the misconceptions that infiltrate this society. I will challenge your preconceptions. I may not change your mind, but I'll do my damnedest to make you think about what you believe. And when you, perhaps, decide you have been narrow-minded about something, I'll offer you an alternate way of looking at things and challenge you to discover your own vision.

So, am I a freak? Yeah, I guess I am in some people's eyes. But I'll continue to be me, no matter what anyone thinks, says, or does. I will always be honest in my work, and I will always be up front as an author, whether through my mysteries or my metaphysical books. I'll wear my Freaks 'R' Us label proudly. I hope you will be true to yourselves and find your own label. Thanks to all of you readers. I sincerely hope that you find something of value in my books. If my experiences can entertain or help you in your own lives, then I'm doing my job.

Bright blessings, and I wish you ecstatic joy in your life.

The Painted Panther
—Yasmine Galenorn

APPENDIX I

Magical Rites and Correspondences

I cover casting a Circle (an area of sacred space) in my book *Embracing the Moon*, but I will present the rudimentary concepts here. The idea behind casting a Circle is to create a sacred space where you can practice your magical workings. When you cast a Circle, you create a space charged with magic that is conducive to spellcraft and ritual. There are many ways to cast a Circle; you should experiment to find which way works best for you. You might find that you vary the way you cast your Circle each time you enter a ritual. It is a good idea to clean your physical space before you enter into magical practice: sweep, clear out cobwebs, clean up clutter. This will help prevent too much chaotic magic filtering into your space.

The simplest and most common method of casting a Circle uses a wand, an athame, a crystal, or your hand, through which you will direct energy. Stand in the center of the room and center yourself. Raise energy through your body and focus it into your hand, or into a tool if you are using one. Channel the energy out of the tool or your hand to create a line of directed force as you slowly turn deosil in a circle, keeping your concentration focused.

You can add chants, you can create an invocation, or you can cast the Circle in silence. I usually cast my Circles thrice: once in the name of the

Young Lord and the Maiden, once in the name of the Father and the Mother, and once in the name of the Sage and the Crone. When you open the Circle, you can use a broom or your hand to sweep the energy away.

Most Witches and Pagans invoke the four elements after they cast a Circle. Together, these elements (Earth, Air, Fire, and Water) create a balance, and together they comprise all life. When we invoke Earth, we invoke the essence of stability, manifestation, abundance, solidity, prosperity, and the physical realm. With Air, we invoke intellect, insight, clarity, and new beginnings. Fire brings us transformation, healing, passion, creativity, and sensuality. With Water, we find emotion, the psyche's hidden depths, introspection, and the ability to adapt.

Elemental Correspondence Tables
The Element of Air

QUALITY	CORRESPONDENCE
Sabbats	Imbolc, Ostara
Direction	East
Realms	The mind—all mental, intellectual, and some psychic work; knowledge; abstract thought; theory; mountaintops; prairie open to the wind; wind; breath; clouds; vapor and mist; storms; purification; removal of stagnation; new beginnings; change
Time	Dawn
Season	Spring
Colors	White, yellow, lavender, pale blue, gray
Zodiac signs	Gemini, Libra, Aquarius
Tools	Censer, incense, athame, sword
Oils	Frankincense, violet, lavender, lemon, rosemary
Faeries	Sylphs
Animals	All birds
Goddesses	Aradia, Arianrhod, Nuit, Urania, Athena
Gods	Mercury, Hermes, Shu, Thoth, Khephera

The Element of Fire

QUALITY	CORRESPONDENCE
Sabbats	Beltane, Litha
Direction	South
Realms	Creativity; passion; energy; blood; healing; destruction; temper; faerie fire, phosphorescence, and will o'the wisps; volcanoes; flame; lava; bonfires; deserts; sun
Time	Noon
Season	Summer
Colors	Red, orange, gold, crimson, peridot, white
Zodiac signs	Leo, Aries, Sagittarius
Tools	Wand, candle
Oils	Lime, orange, neroli, citronella
Faeries	Flame Dancers, Phoenix
Animals	Salamander, snake, lizard
Goddesses	Pele, Freyja, Vesta, Hestia, Brighid
Gods	Vulcan, Horus, Ra, Agni, Hephaestus

The Element of Water

QUALITY	CORRESPONDENCE
Sabbats	Lughnasadh, Mabon
Direction	West
Realms	Emotions; feelings; love; sorrow; intuition; the subconscious and unconscious minds; the womb; fertility; menstruation; cleansing; purification; oceans; lakes; tidepools; rain; springs and wells
Time	Afternoon
Season	Autumn
Colors	Blue, blue gray, aquamarine, lavender, white, gray, indigo, royal purple

QUALITY	CORRESPONDENCE
Zodiac signs	Pisces, Scorpio, Cancer
Tools	Chalice, cauldron
Oils	Lemon, lily of the valley, camphor
Faeries	Naiads, Undines, Sirens
Animals	All fish and marine life
Goddesses	Aphrodite, Isis, Mari, Tiamat, Vellamo, Ran, Kupala
Gods	Ahto, Osiris, Manannan, Neptune, Poseidon, Varuna

The Element of Earth

QUALITY	CORRESPONDENCE
Sabbats	Samhain, Yule
Direction	North
Realms	The body; growth; nature; sustenance; material gain; prosperity; money; death; caverns; fields; meadows; plants; trees; animals; rocks; crystals; manifestation; materialization
Time	Midnight
Season	Winter
Colors	Black, brown, green, gold, mustard
Zodiac signs	Capricorn, Taurus, Virgo
Tools	Pentacle
Oils	Pine, cypress, cedar, sage, vetiver
Faeries	Paras, Kobolds, Dwarves
Animals	All four-footed animals
Goddesses	Ceres, Demeter, Gaia, Persephone, Kore, Rhea, Epona, Cerridwen
Gods	Cernunnos, Herne, Dionysus, Marduk, Pan, Tammuz, Attis, Thor, Tapio

Simple Circle Casting and Invocation of the Elements

In the center of your ritual space, stand with your dagger (or tool of choice). Focus on drawing energy through you and directing it into your blade. Circle slowly from north, deosil (clockwise), three times. Say:

I cast this Circle once in the name of the Young Lord and the Maiden.

I cast this Circle twice in the name of the Father and the Mother.

I cast this Circle thrice in the name of the Sage and the Crone.

Turn to the north, and say:

I invoke thee, Spirits of the Earth, you who are bone and stone and crystal, you who are rock and tree and branch and leaf. I invoke thee, you who are deepest caverns to the highest mountaintops. Come to me and bring with you your stability, your manifestation, your abundance and prosperity. Come to these rites, Spirits of Earth. Welcome and Blessed Be.

Turn to the east, and say:

I invoke thee, Spirits of the Wind, you who are the chill breeze, you who are mist and fog and vapor and the gale of the hurricane. I invoke thee, you who are the rising winds and the gentle calm. Come to me and bring with you your keen insight and clarity of mind, sweep through and remove stagnation and bring new beginnings. Come to these rites, Spirits of Wind. Welcome and Blessed Be.

Turn to the south, and say:

I invoke thee, Spirits of Flame, you who are the crackling bonfire, you who are warmth of the hearth, the golden glow of the sun through the forest at midday. I invoke thee, you who are the glowing lava and the heat of the desert sands. Come to me and bring with you your passion and creativity, your healing and transformation. Come to these rites, Spirits of Flame. Welcome and Blessed Be.

Turn to the west, and say:

I invoke thee, Spirits of the Water, you who are the raging river, you who are the crashing ocean breakers and the still pool of the grotto. I invoke thee, you who are the tears of our body, the rain kissing our brow. Come to me and bring with you joy and sorrow, laughter and tears, peace and enthusiasm. Lead me into the hidden depths of my psyche and guide the way into my heart. Come to these rites, Spirits of Water. Welcome and Blessed Be.

Devoking the Elements and Opening the Circle

When the ritual is over, you will probably want to devoke the elements and open the Circle. This will open the energy pathways. Occasionally I leave a Circle intact, to settle into the walls of the house.

Turn to the west, and say:

Spirits of the Water, Spirits of the Ocean, thank you for attending our Circle. Go if you must, stay if you will. Hail and Farewell.

Turn to the south, and say:

Spirits of Flame, Spirits of the Fire, thank you for attending our Circle. Go if you must, stay if you will. Hail and Farewell.

Turn to the east, and say:

Spirits of the Wind, Spirits of the Air, thank you for attending our Circle. Go if you must, stay if you will. Hail and Farewell.

Turn to the north, and say:

> *Spirits of the Earth, Spirits of the Mountains, thank you for attending our Circle. Go if you must, stay if you will. Hail and Farewell.*

Take your broom, or use your hand, and slowly turn widdershins while envisioning the ring of energy opening. If you cast the Circle thrice, then devoke it with three turns; if you cast it once, then devoke it with one turn. Say:

> *This Circle is open but unbroken.*

> *Merry Meet, Merry Part, and Merry Meet again!*

Smudging

Smudging is the act of using smoke to cleanse energy or an aura. You can use either a stick of incense, some granular incense on charcoal designed for this purpose, or a smudge stick (usually a bundle of sage, or sage and lavender, or sweetgrass). Make sure sparks don't fly onto clothing, and don't hold the smudge stick too close to someone's skin. Also be considerate enough to ask whether people have allergies before you light up incense.

Drawing Down Position

This position seems to be advantageous for opening the aura and body in order to receive energy from outside oneself. Stand with your legs separated, your feet firmly planted on the floor. Keep your back comfortably straight and your chin up, and gaze toward the ceiling. Your arms may be extended out to the side, palms up in a receiving position, or you may bend your elbows at your sides, with your palms open and facing the ceiling.

Moon and Sun Water

Moon water is water that has been charged under the moon's energy. Sun water is water that has been charged by the light of the sun. Both are used in magical rites and spells, depending on what energy is needed.

Full Moon Water

Fill a glass jar with water. Add a moonstone to the jar, and cap it. Three days before a full moon, set the jar outside at night where it can capture the moon's rays (it doesn't matter if it is overcast). Bring the jar in the following morning. Repeat this for the next two nights. After this, add water each month as needed, setting the jar outside the night before the full moon.

New Moon Water

Fill a glass jar with water. Add a piece of black onyx to the jar, and cap it. Follow the directions as above, but set the jar outside during the new moon (and three days before it), instead of the time of the full moon.

Sun Water

Fill a glass jar with water. Add a piece of citrine or carnelian to the jar, and cap it. Set the jar outside on three consecutive sunny days, taking the jar inside at dusk. For added strength, set the jar outside at dawn on the morning of the summer solstice. Use sun water for solar rituals and spells.

Resources

Music for Rituals and Meditations

BAND	TITLE
Gabrielle Roth and The Mirrors:	*Tongues, Totem, Bones, Ritual, Initiation, Endless Wave, Waves, Luna, Zone Unknown*
Dead Can Dance:	*Into the Labyrinth, Spiritchaser, Aion, The Serpent's Egg*
Mike Oldfield:	*Tubular Bells*
Phil Thorntan and Hossam Ramsy:	*Eternal Egypt*
Suvarna:	*Fire of the Oracle*

Videotapes

Kama Sutra: A Tale of Love:	1997, directed by Mira Nair, rated R. A spectacular love story set in sixteenth century India; incredible photography; brilliant settings and haunting eye candy; erotica.
Aria	1987. Ten vignettes based on operatic drama; erotica.

Online Sites

Online sites come and go. If you do not find a site that is listed here, don't contact me about it. But you might try a search on the name to see whether it has moved to a new URL.

General Magic

Circle Sanctuary: www.circlesanctuary.org
Galenorn En/Visions: www.galenorn.com
Gothic Gardening: www.gothic.net/~malice
JBL Statues: sacredsource.com
Mystical Grove, A: www.amysticalgrove.com
New Moon Rising: www.nmrising.com (see also "Magical Magazines")
Nine Houses of Gaia, The: www.9houses.org
Raven's World: www.ravensworld.com (see also "Magical Supplies")
Wiccan-Pagan Times, The: www.twpt.com
Widdershins: www.widdershins.org (see also "Magical Magazines")
Witch's Brew: www.witchs-brew.com
Witches Voice, The: www.witchvox.com

BDSM

Bedroom Bondage: www.bedroombondage.com
Different Loving: www.gloria-brame.com
DungeonNet.com: www.dungeons.net
Kinky Cards: www.kinkycards.com
Meretrix Online: www.realm-of-shade.com/meretrix
Wet Spot, The: www.wetspot.org

Polyamory

Church of All Worlds: www.caw.org
Loving More: www.lovemore.com
Polyamory Society, The: www.polyamorysociety.org

Tantra and Sacred Sex

Goddess Temple, The: www.goddesstemple.com

Sacred Sex: www.luckymojo.com/sacredsex.html

TantraWorks: www.tantraworks.com

Yoga Tantra Veda: www.geocities.com/Athens/Olympus/3588/
yotaveda.html

Sex Toys

Adult Toy Chest: adulttoychest.com

Good Vibrations: www.goodvibes.com

Lovers Package: www.loverspackage.com

Toys in Babeland: www.babeland.com

Gay and Lesbian Resources

Kurfew Club: www.kurfew.com

Pflag: www.pflag.org

Ten Percent Bent: www.tenpercentbent.com

BBW Connections for Big Beautiful Women

BBW Magazine: www.bbwmagazine.com (P.O. Box 1297, Elk Grove,
CA 95759)

Dimensions OnLine: www.pencomputing.com/dim

NAAFA: www.naafa.org (P.O. Box 188620, Sacramento, CA 95818;
phone: 916-558-6880; fax: 916-558-6881)

Radiance Magazine: www.radiancemagazine.com (P.O. Box 30246,
Oakland, CA 94604; phone: 510-482-0680; fax: 510-482-1576)

Activists

ACLU: www.aclu.org

Interfaith Alliance, The: www.interfaithalliance.org

National Civil Rights Museum, The: www.civilrightsmuseum.org

National Organization for Women: www.now.org

Magical Supplies

Most of the shops listed here offer mail order and/or online service and catalogs. However, retail shops go in and out of business with alarming frequency, and web-based businesses can have an even briefer existence. So some shops listed may not be in service when you write to them.

As for local supplies, look for candles in drug stores, stationery stores, grocery stores, and gift shops. Grocery stores and florists carry flowers, as do your friends' gardens. You can sometimes find essential oils in gift shops or perfume shops, and gift shops and rock shops may carry crystals. Gather your herbs wild or purchase them in grocery stores, food co-ops, herb shops, or local plant nurseries (the plant itself).

Unusual altar pieces can often be found at local import stores and secondhand stores. Altar cloths are easy; go to your favorite fabric shop and buy a piece of cloth large enough to cover your altar table.

Don't overlook the Yellow Pages. Look under Metaphysical, Herbs, Books (bookstores often carry much more than just books), Lapidary Supplies, and Jewelry.

Azure Green
48-WEB
Middlefield, MA 01243-0048
(413) 623-2155

White Light Pentacles
P.O. Box 8163
Salem, MA 01971-8163
(978) 745-8668 or (978) 741-2355

Serpentine Music Productions
P.O. Box 2564
Sebastopol, CA 95473
(707) 823-7425
(carries a wide variety of hard-to-find pagan music)

Gypsy Heaven
115G South Main Street
New Hope, PA 18938
(215) 862-5251

Moon Scents
P.O. Box 1109
North Conway, NH 03860
(603) 356-3666

Edge of the Circle Books
701 E. Pike
Seattle, WA 98122
(206) 726-1999

Raven's World
15600 NE 8th Street
Bellevue, WA 98008
(425) 644-7502

JBL Statues
Sacred Source / JBL
P.O. Box WW
Crozet, VA 22932-0163
Phone: (800) 290-6203
Phone: (804) 823-1515
Fax: (804) 823-7665
Email: spirit@sacredsource.com

Magical Magazines

Beltane Papers, The
P.O. Box 29694
Bellingham, WA 98228-1694

New Moon Rising
P.O. Box 1731
Medford, OR 97501-0135
(541) 858-9404
Fax: (541) 779-8815

Open Ways
P.O. Box 87704
Vancouver, WA 98687

SageWoman
P.O. Box 641
Point Arena, CA 95648
(707) 882-2052

Shaman's Drum
P.O. Box 97
Ashland, OR 97520

Widdershins
Emerald City/Silver Moon Productions
12345 Lake City Way NE, Suite 268
Seattle, WA 98125

Glossary

AIDS. Acquired immune deficiency syndrome, caused by an HIV infection. A complex syndrome of symptoms usually leading to death.

Altar. The ritual layout of magical and ritual tools and symbols.

Athame. A ritual dagger, usually double-bladed.

Aura. The energy field existing around all living things.

Autoerotism. Erotic self-pleasuring.

BDSM. Bondage, domination, and sadomasochism. The practices of pain and pleasure, of sexual domination and restriction. These practices have been around since the beginning of time, but they are only a somewhat acceptable practice.

Beltane. A pagan celebration of life and sexuality that occurs on May 1.

Bilocation. The ability to be in two places at once.

Bisexual. A person who is sexually attracted to either gender.

Bottom. A person who is the passive partner during sexual play, though not necessarily submissive.

Bower. An outdoor boudoir specifically set aside as a retreat where couples can make love.

Censer. An incense burner.

Centering. The act of finding an internal point of balance.

Cervix. The opening at the bottom of the uterus that dilates to allow babies to emerge from the womb.

Chalice. A ritual goblet.

Chlamydia. A sexually transmitted disease that can result in sterility.

Circle. A sphere constructed of energy, created by a Witch. A sacred space.

Cleansing. The act of removing negative energy or purifying.

Clitoris. The tiny bud that is the chief sexual pleasure center for women, analogous to the penis in men.

Contraception. A barrier to conceiving.

Craft. Witchcraft, the practice of natural magic.

Crone. The aged aspect of the Goddess, representing wisdom, experience, and the Underworld.

Deosil. Clockwise (sunwise) direction.

Dominant. A male dominator during sexual play. Also called *dom*.

Dominatrix. A female dominator during sexual play. Also called *domina* or *domme*.

Elements. The four building blocks of the universe—Earth, Air, Fire, and Water. Major forces used in natural magic.

Equinox, autumnal. The point during autumn when the sun crosses the celestial equator, and day and night are of equal length. See Mabon.

Equinox, vernal. The point during spring when the sun crosses the celestial equator, and day and night are of equal length. See Ostara.

Faggot. A term for gay men, often used in a derogatory fashion. Also used by some number of gay men to reclaim the word. The term refers to the fact that homosexuals were burned at the stake during the Inquisition, like faggots for a fire. Also called a *fag*.

Fag hag. A woman who hangs out with or is attracted to gay men.

Fallopian tube. The tube the egg passes through on its way from the ovary to the uterus.

Gay. A man who is sexually attracted to other men.

Gonorrhea. A sexually transmitted disease, which, if left untreated, can lead to sterility and can damage the reproductive organs.

Great Rite. The union of a man and a woman to symbolize the union of the God and Goddess, usually enacted by a Priest and Priestess. The Great Rite can be actual or symbolic.

Green Man. A male aspect of divinity symbolized by vegetation and forests. Also called *Jack-in-the-Green.*

Ground. To root oneself firmly in the physical world in preparation for magical or metaphysical work.

Hepatitis C. An infection that can be sexually transmitted. It has no known cure and can lead to chronic hepatitis and increased risks for liver cancer.

Herpes. A sexually transmitted disease that is incurable. It is an ongoing problem for many of its carriers and victims.

Heterosexual. A person who is sexually attracted to the opposite gender.

Hieros Gamos. Formal term for the Divine Marriage between the Goddess and her Consort-God or their earthly representatives.

HIV. A human immunodeficiency virus that leads to the acquired immune deficiency syndrome (AIDS).

Houris. Sacred harlots (Persian) and/or Priestesses of the Goddess.

HPV. Human papillomavirus, a sexually transmitted disease that can lead to increased risks of genital cancer in both sexes.

Hunt. The Wild Hunt led by (various) gods and/or goddesses.

Hunter. The Horned God of the Witches.

Imbola. The Pagan celebration of the Goddess Brighid, celebrated on February 2nd.

Invocation. An appeal or petition to a god or goddess, element, or energy.

Jack-in-the-Green. See Green Man.

Kegel exercises. Exercises designed to strengthen the sexual muscles.

King Stag. See Stag King.

Kink. Kink is the more positive way of referring to a sexual practice not generally accepted as normal. Also referred to as *perversion*, which carries a negative connotation.

Labia majora. Two folds of fatty tissue that extend from the mons veneris back between the legs.

Labia minora. The tissue that surrounds the vaginal opening.

Lesbian. A woman who is sexually attracted to other women.

Litha. The Pagan celebration of summer solstice.

Lughnasadh. The Pagan celebration of the First Harvest (the harvest of grain) celebrated on August 1st.

Mabon. The Pagan celebration of the autumnal equinox.

Magic. The manipulation of natural forces and psychic energy to bring about desired changes. Also referred to as Magick by many Pagans.

Maiden. The youthful aspect of the Goddess, representing freedom, adventure, and playfulness.

Masturbation. See Autoerotism.

Maypole. A tree or long pole used for dances during Beltane, representing the phallus of the God. See Beltane.

May Queen. A representative of the Goddess, she rules over Beltane and is associated with the Stag King.

Meditation. A state of reflection or contemplation.

Menstrual cycle. The cycle of menstruation.

Menstruation. The shedding of blood and lining when an unfertilized egg passes through a woman's uterus.

Monogamy. A one-to-one sexual relationship between two persons of any gender. Practitioners believe that an exclusive sexual commitment deepens love and trust.

Mother. The fertile, full-grown aspect of the Goddess, representing the prime of life, creativity, and adult sexuality.

Orgasm. A sexual climax or peak.

Ostara. The Pagan celebration of the vernal equinox.

Ovaries. Female organs that produce eggs that may become embryos.

Ovulation. The time when an egg ripens, releasing from the ovaries and passing into the uterus.

Pagan. A follower of one of many ancient and/or modern revivals of Earth-centered religions.

Panfidelity. The belief that one can and should sexually connect with anyone they feel a bond with (as long as it's reciprocal). The panfidelitist usually espouses no permanent or long-term relationships unless they are sexually open.

Penis. The major male sexual organ, extending two to four inches when flaccid and five to seven inches when erect. It is used for urination as well as sexual intercourse.

Polarity. The concept of equal, opposite energies.

Polyamory. A group relationship or marriage, usually founded on basic rules that the group of lovers bind themselves to. New lovers generally are not taken in without the approval of all members. The polyamorist tends to believe that no one person can meet all of another persons needs.

Prostate. The male gland that surrounds the urethra at the bladder.

RAINN. The Rape, Abuse, and Incest National Network, founded by Tori Amos.

Rape. A crime of violence, which uses sex as a weapon to degrade, humiliate, and control.

Ritual. A ceremony.

Ritualist. One who takes part in a ritual.

Runes. Symbols that are carved onto rocks, crystals, or clay, which embody powerful energies to be used during magical practices. They are also symbols used in early alphabets.

Sabbat. Any of the eight pagan holidays that comprise the Wheel of the Year.

Sacred harlot. A woman who offers her sexuality to others in a sacred and reverent manner. This can also refer to a priestess of a goddess of sexuality.

Safe, Sane, and Consensual. This refers to sex play that does not unduly endanger anyone, that both (or all) partners agree on, and that is kept within the bounds of the agreed-upon rules.

Samhain. The pagan celebration honoring the dead, celebrated on November 1st.

Scrotum. The sac below the penis that holds the testes or testicles.

Semen. Seminal fluid transports the sperm into the vagina.

Sex magick. The use of sexual energy and play to focus and work magic.

Sexual communion. Communion with the divine through sexual play.

Sheelah Na Gig. A figure carved in stone, depicting a woman spreading her genitals wide, pandemic in Europe and the United Kingdom and thought to represent women's sacred sexuality or perhaps the Goddess herself.

Smudge. The act of purifying or cleansing the air through the use of smoke. See Smudge Stick.

Smudge stick. A bundle of herbs used for smudging. See Smudging.

Sperm. The male fluid of fertility. Also called *spermatozoa.*

Stag King. The symbol of the Horned God in Celtic beliefs. It is also seen as a symbol for the rightful ruler of the land. The Stag King, or King Stag, is a white stag, which is very rare and sacred.

Submissive. A person who is submissive during sexual play. Also called a *sub* or a *bottom.*

Syphilis. A sexually transmitted disease that can, if untreated, lead to madness, blindness, and eventual death.

Tantra. A Hindu practice of sacred sexuality.

Testes. See Testicles.

Testicles. The external organ on men that produces sperm.

Top. A person who is the active partner during sexual play, but is not necessarily dominant.

Tradition. A specific subgroup of Pagans, Witches, Wiccans, or magic workers.

Uterus. The womb, the receptacle in which the fertilized egg may grow into a fetus and a full-term baby.

Vagina. The internal sheath of flesh through which a baby passes at birth, through which menstrual fluid passes, and into which the male inserts his penis during sexual intercourse.

Vanilla people. People who generally enjoy straight sex with no kinks, who are heterosexual, and who are usually in monogamous relationships.

Vanilla sex. Straight sex with no kinks.

Visualization. The process of forming mental images.

Wheel of the Year. The cyclic turn of the seasons.

Widdershins. Counterclockwise.

Witch. A practitioner of the craft of magic, or Witchcraft, usually also a member of a Pagan religion.

Yuletide. The Pagan celebration of the winter solstice.

Bibliography

Anand, Margo. *The Art of Sexual Ecstasy.* Los Angeles: Jeremy P. Tarcher, Inc., 1989.

Anderson, William, and Clive Hicks. *Green Man.* London & New York: HarperCollins, 1990.

Arons, Katie, with Jacqueline Shannon. *Sexy at Any Size.* New York: Fireside Books, 1999.

Barbach, Lonnie. *The Erotic Edge.* New York: Plume Books, 1996.

———. *For Yourself: The Fulfillment of Female Sexuality.* New York: Signet Books, 1975.

———. *Pleasures: Women Write Erotica.* New York: Harper Perennial, 1984.

Block, Joel D. *Secrets to Better Sex.* West Nyack, NY: Parker Publishing, 1996.

Brame, Gloria G., William D. Brame, and Jon Jacobs. *Different Loving: The World of Sexual Dominance and Submission.* New York: Villard, 1993.

Campbell, Joseph. *The Masks of God: Occidental Mythology.* New York: Penguin, 1991.

Chu, Valentin. *The Yin-Yang Butterfly.* New York: Jeremy P. Tarcher/Putnam, 1993.

Conway, D.J. *Lord of Light and Shadow.* St. Paul, MN: Llewellyn Worldwide, 1997.

———. *The Ancient and Shining Ones.* St. Paul, MN: Llewellyn Worldwide, 1993.

Debetz, Barbara, and Samm Sinclair Baker. *Erotic Focus*. New York: Signet Books, 1986.

Dunas, Felice. *Passion Play*. New York: Riverhead Books, 1997.

Farrar, Janet and Stewart. *The Witches' Goddess*. Custer, WA: Phoenix Publishing, Inc., 1987.

———. *The Witches' God*. Custer, WA: Phoenix Publishing, Inc., 1989.

———. *Forbidden Flowers*. New York: Pocket Books, 1975.

———. *Men in Love*. New York: Dell Publishing, 1980.

Friday, Nancy. *My Secret Garden: Women's Sexual Fantasies*. New York: Pocket Books, 1973.

———. *Women on Top: How Real Life Has Changed Women's Sexual Fantasies*. New York: Simon & Schuster, 1991.

———. *Crafting the Body Divine*. Santa Cruz, CA: The Crossing Press, 2001.

———. *Dancing with the Sun*. St. Paul, MN: Llewellyn Worldwide, 1999.

Galenorn, Yasmine. *Embracing the Moon*. St. Paul, MN: Llewellyn Worldwide, 1998.

———. *Tarot Journeys*. St. Paul, MN: Llewellyn Worldwide, 1999.

———. *Trancing the Witch's Wheel*. St. Paul, MN: Llewellyn Worldwide, 1997.

Graham-Maw, Jane. *Kama Sutra: The Arts of Love*. San Francisco: Thorsons, 1992.

Grahn, Judy. *Another Mother Tongue*. Boston: Beacon Press, 1994.

Graves, Robert. *The White Goddess: A Historical Grammar of Poetic Myth*. Gloucester, MA: Peter Smith Publisher, Inc., 1983.

Hunt, Morton. *The Natural History of Love*. New York: Anchor Books, 1994.

Hutchins, Loraine, and Lani Kaahumanu. *Bi Any Other Name*. Boston: Alyson Publications, 1991.

Lubell, Winifred Milius. *The Metamorphosis of Baubo*. Nashville and London: Vanderbilt University Press, 1994.

Mac Cana, Proinsias. *Celtic Mythology*. London: Hamlyn, 1970.

MacLean, Helene. *EveryWoman's Health*. New York: Doubleday Book and Music Clubs, Inc., 1980.

Miller, Philip, and Molly Devon. *Screw the Roses, Send Me the Thorns*. Fairfield, CT: Mystic Books, 1995.

Neel, Alexandra David. *Magic and Mystery in Tibet*. New York: Dover Publications, Inc., 1971.

Raley, Patricia. *Making Love*. New York: Avon Books, 1976.

Reese, Laura. *Topping from Below*. New York: St. Martin's Press, 1995.

Sinha, Indra. *The Great Book of Tantra*. Rochester, VT: Destiny Books, 1993.

Sprenger, James, and Heinrich Kramer. *Malleus Maleficarum*. 1486. Translated by Montague Summers. London: John Rodker, 1928.

Stewart, Jessica. *The Complete Manual of Sexual Positions*. Chatworth, CA: Media Press, 1983.

Stone, Merlin. When God Was a Woman, New York: Harcourt Brace/Harvest Books, 1978.

Westheimer, Ruth. *Ruth's Guide to Good Sex*. New York: Warner Books, 1983.

I also wish to cite these Internet sites that I used in my research:

Bieda, Jessica. "Women in Mesopotamia." University of Arizona.

California State University Northridge. "Aphrodite (Inanna)."

Encyclopedia Britannica Online.

Halsall, Paul. "Homosexual Eros in Early Greece." Fordham University.

Internet Classics Archives. "The Deeds of the Divine Augustus."

Konstan, David. "Materials for the Study of Women and Gender in the Ancient World—Women, Ethnicity and Power in the Roman Empire." www.stoa.org.

Lefkowitz, Mary, and Maureen Fant. "Materials for the Study of Women and Gender in the Ancient World—Legal Status in the Roman World." www.stoa.org.

Snook, Jennifer. "The Perseus Project: Sappho's Legacy."

Index

G

Galenorn, Jasmine, xii, 65, 80, 118, 137, 145, 237
Gems
  citrine, 71
  diamonds, 77
  emeralds, 72
  of Gods/Goddesses, 228–230
  jacinth, 70
  rubies, 68, 69
  sapphires, 74
Genital mutilation, 19
Gods and Goddesses
  described, 227–231
  invoking, 102–103, 121, 160, 231
  pagan beliefs about, 117
  sexual partner as, 140
  sexual polarity of, 186
  See also specific Gods and Goddesses
Golden showers, 47
Gonorrhea, 29, 257
Great Rite, 95, 99, 165–166, 168–170, 257
  See also Hieros Gamos
Greece, 4–5
Green Man, 96, 116, 117, 257
  See also Stag King
Group marriage, 191–192
"G spot," 26
Guilt
  fantasies and, 90–91
  overcoming, 57, 208–209
  sex and, 52–53

H

Hammurabi, 2
Har. *See* Ishtar
Hate crimes, 184
  See also Rape
Hathor rune, 79
Henkin, Bill, 65
Hepatitis C, 30, 257
Herbal charms, 81
Hermaphrodite, 186
Herne, 116, 118, 121, 126–131, 135
Herpes, 29, 257
Hetaerae, 4–5

Hieros Gamos, 95, 165–168, 257
  See also Great Rite
History of sexuality, 1–20
  Christianity, 8–15
  courtly love, 15–16
  Greece, 4–5
  Puritans, 16–17
  restoration period, 17
  Rome, 5–7
  Sumer to Judea, 2–4
  Twentieth Century, 19–20
  Victorian era, 17–19
Hitchhiking, 203
HIV/AIDS, 28–29, 30, 255, 257
Homosexuality
  acceptance exercise, 183–185
  attitudes toward, 182–183
  Christianity and, 10
  Divine Communion and, 99
  fantasies about, 92–93
  fear of, 62–63, 173–174
  Goddess of, 186
  sex magic and, 185–186
  stereotyping, 182
  websites, 250
  See also Artemis ritual; Pan ritual
HPV (human papillomavirus), 30, 257
Humiliation, 208
Hunter Gods
  Cernunnos, 116, 118, 121
  Herne, 116, 118, 121, 126–131, 135
  See also Stag King
Hunting Lord Oil, 137
Hygiene, 87

I

Incest, 211–212
Innocent VIII, Pope, 11–13
Inquisition, 11–15
Insomnia, 209
Intoxication Oil Version #2, 114
Ishtar, 97, 102–103, 229
  See also Sacred Harlot

K

Kali-Ma, 98, 229
Kama Sutra, 156, 157

269

W

X, Y, Z